Stroke Prevention

Stroke Prevention

Editors
Wolfgang Dorndorf, Giessen
Peter Marx, Berlin

26 figures and 29 tables, 1994

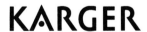

Basel · Freiburg · Paris · London · New York · New Delhi · Bangkok · Singapore · Tokyo · Sydney

Library of Congress Cataloging-in-Publication Data

International Symposium on Stroke Prevention (1992 : Berlin, Germany)
Stroke prevention / International Symposium on Stroke Prevention,
Berlin, April 12–14, 1992 ; editors: Wolfgang Dorndorf, Peter Marx.
Includes bibliographical references and index.
ISBN 3-8055-5882-1 (alk. paper)
1. Cerebrovascular disease-Prevention-Congresses. I. Dorndorf, Wolfgang. II. Marx, Peter,
1937–. III. Title.
[DNLM: 1. Cerebrovascular Disorders-prevention & control-congresses. 2. Cerebrovascular
Disorders-etiology-congresses. 3. Risk Factors-congresses. WL 355 I6045s 1992]
RC388.5.I5159 1992
616.8'1-dc20
DNLM/DLC for Library of Congress   93-38418 CIP

Drug Dosage
The authors and the publisher have exerted every effort to ensure that drug selection and dosage set forth in this text are in accord with current recommendations and practice at the time
of publication. However, in view of ongoing research, changes in government regulations,
and the constant flow of information relating to drug therapy and drug reactions, the reader is
urged to check the package insert for each drug for any change in indications and dosage and
for added warnings and precautions. This is particularly important when the recommended
agent is a new and/or infrequently employed drug.

© Copyright 1994 by S. Karger GmbH, Postfach, D-79095 Freiburg, and
S. Karger AG, P. O. Box, CH-4009 Basel
Printed in Germany by Konkordia Druck GmbH, D-77815 Bühl
ISBN 3-8055-5882-1

Contents

Contents

Surgical and Interventional Prevention

Cardioembolic Stroke

Preface

Despite growing knowledge about the pathophysiology of cerebral ischemia and great efforts to find rational therapies, stroke treatment is still not very effective, leaving many survivors chronically disabled.

In contrast to the scanty results of stroke treatment, stroke prevention is quite efficacious in hypertensive patients and those with atrial fibrillation and severe symptomatic carotid stenosis. Based on knowledge about risk factors and improved methods to identify stroke etiologies in individual patients, various interventional studies have been initiated and proved that stroke can be avoided in a considerable number of patients.

In order to give a summary of state of the art science in this field and also to discuss future developments, an International Symposium on Stroke Prevention was held in Berlin in April 1992. Leading scientists from Europe and abroad discussed issues such as Etiological Classification of Stroke, Risk Factor Evaluation, Secondary Prevention in Vascular Disease, Surgical and Interventional Prevention, and Prevention of Cardioembolic Stroke. The results of this meeting are presented in this book.

The editors are indebted to all participants who contributed to this publication.

Wolfgang Dorndorf
Peter Marx

Classification

Dorndorf W, Marx P (eds): Stroke Prevention.
Basel, Karger, 1994, pp 1–13

Classification of Strokes: Experience from Stroke Data Banks

J. P. Mohr

Neurological Institute, Columbia-Presbyterian Medical Center, New York, N.Y., USA

The advancement of technologies to image the brain and blood vessels, by such methods as CT, MR, duplex and transcranial Doppler, and SPECT, has greatly assisted attempts to create a reliable stroke diagnosis algorithm. In the past, the determination of infarct subtype was mainly made on clinical grounds and based on the clinical syndrome and coexisting risk factors. The rare autopsy confirmation provided only a small data base to check the accuracy of the algorithm and other diagnostic studies; the clinical impressions have been refined and supported by laboratory confirmation of the infarct subtype.

A large data base can be put to many uses, from discovery of the role of risk factors [1], to the use of imaging technologies [2], detection of unusual forms of stroke, insights into pathophysiology [3], preparation for clinical trials [4], diagnosis to prognosis [5–8], inter-institutional comparison [9], to name but a few. This article is mainly concerned with issues of diagnosis of stroke subtype.

Problems in Clinical and Laboratory Diagnosis of Hemorrhage

Parenchymatous hemorrhage is no longer an issue in diagnosis, especially in the acute phase within days of onset, when CT or MR imaging is available. The outcome can be predicted when the data base is large enough [10]. The prognosis for survival seems to be related to the location as well as to the size of the hematoma [11].

Thanks to good-quality MR scanning, cavernous angiomas and small arteriovenous malformations are now capable of being diagnosed and separated from other sources of brain hemorrhage.

Cavernous angiomas usually show a distinctive central focus of high signal surrounded by hypointensity on MR, which was initially considered pathognomonic for cavernous angiomas but no longer is so. Small arteriovenous malformations have yielded the same appearance as have small primary hemorrhages, so the picture should be considered mainly that of small hematoma from any cause.

Prior to the availability of high-quality brain imaging, the diagnosis of hemorrhage rested on the finding of blood in the spinal fluid or of a major mass effect on angiogram. Yet small, deep hematomas usually do not reach the ventricular wall, and the spinal fluid is clear. Large avascular masses could have many origins, hemorrhage among them, but tumor, abscess, encephalitis, and the like are other possibilities not ruled out by the angiogram.

When CT is not available, a differentiation of hemorrhage from infarction remains a bit difficult on clinical grounds alone. Studies developing models for discriminators rely on decreased consciousness, headache, nausea and vomiting as predictors of hemorrhage [12]. Highly circumscribed focal deficits from small lesions, whether from hemorrhage or from infarction, can easily mislead those relying on the clinical syndrome alone to mistakenly diagnose infarction. No reliable clinical criteria have been established to separate these syndromes of small lesions except that Wallenberg's lateral medullary syndrome has thus far not been reported from hematoma. All other focal eponymic syndromes have had at least a few case reports from hematoma, including all the syndromes thought due to 'lacunes' such as pure motor stroke, ataxic hemiparesis, pure sensory stroke; circumscribed speech and language disorders such as dyspraxia from a lesion in Broca's area, pure word deafness, pure alexia, and ideomotor dyspraxia from a callosal lesion.

Hemorrhagic infarction remains a difficult differential diagnosis based on brain imaging alone [13].

Problems in Clinical and Laboratory Diagnosis of Infarction

Algorithms for classification of the ischemic stroke by infarct subtype have greatly improved but still remains difficult. On clinical grounds alone, the traditional use of age, risk factors, and mode of onset are used to try and separate embolism from thrombosis, under the assumption that embolism carries a risk of recurrence not seen from thrombosis and that surgery could apply for thrombosis but not for embolism. Neither of these viewpoints apply any longer. Embolism can occur from thrombotic lesions and surgery can be a means of removing a source of embolism [14]. Both forms of ischemic stroke have a high frequency of recurrence, although the lacunar syndromes seem to have the lowest. One major reason for seeking a diagnosis of thrombosis is to seek evidence of high-grade carotid stenosis which might be amenable to prophylactic carotid endarterectomy. MR angiography has been an important new development because it provides opportunities to look for arterial dissections not easily found by duplex Doppler.

Few studies have collected detailed information on the clinical and radiologic characteristics of large homogeneous subsets of patients with acute cerebral infarction. The Stroke Data Bank provided a large collection of prospectively collected information on patients with different subtypes of infarction. A deliberate attempt was made to classify patients into distinct categories and create new subsets based on presumed mechanism of infarction. This effort resulted in some changes in the large categories of stroke due to infarction. In particular, the group often labeled as atherothrombosis was divided into two subgroups: large artery thrombosis with no evidence of embolic infarction and a form of artery-to-artery embolism arising from an atherosclerotic source. A separate category, infarct of undetermined cause, was created to help insure the homogenity of the Stroke Data Bank diagnostic groups.

Despite these efforts, in a disappointingly high percentage of cases, no diagnosis as to exact mechanism of infarction was reached. It became apparent that many cases were diagnosed on the 'best clinical guess'. Where laboratory data was available, the results indicated that large artery atherosclerotic occlusive disease was a less frequent cause of stroke; small vessel or lacunar and cardioembolic infarction were relatively frequent; and that the cause for the majority of the cases of infarction could not be classified into these traditional diagnostic categories. The large frequency of surface infarcts in the setting of a normal or distal branch arterial occlusion led most to consider these unexplained cerebral infarcts as examples of embolism where the thrombotic source was undetected. Our findings have forced the creation of a separate diagnostic category for cases whose mechanisms of infarction remain unproven, one known as 'infarct of undetermined cause' or 'cryptogenic infarction'. Apart from a few features they share in common, this category of infarction remains poorly understood and, as yet, has not been successfully characterized as a clinical group.

Cryptogenic Infarction (Infarct of Undetermined Cause)

Many explanations exist for lack of a definitive diagnosis of infarct mechanism can be offered. The usual is that no studies were performed, or those done were the wrong ones. Given a major stroke in a person of advanced age with coexisting severe disease, many physicians are simply unwilling to undertake further tests. These are only a few of the many reasons for deferring a workup. When testing is done, there is often a problem in timing: emboli are known to disappear within hours to days and may be gone if the imaging studies are delayed too long, leaving the CT or MR signs of infarction but with normal vessels.

Despite all the excuses, as many as 40% of cases of ischemic stroke fail to have the mechanism clarified. Emerging technologies have shown that some of these cases may be explained by hematologic disorders causing hypercoagulable states from protein C, free protein S [15], lupus anticoagulant or anticardiolipin antibody abnormalities. The numbers seem to be small but the exact frequencies remain unsettled [16]. One recent development has been the documentation of a surprisingly high frequency of paradoxical emboli through a patent cardiac foramen ovale [17]. Arteritis seems rare enough that it will remain a tiny fraction of the cases of cryptogenic stroke. Of unknown frequency is spontaneous vasospasm, such as is inferred to occur in migraine, affecting arteries with enough severity to cause infarction.

Adding up all the causes of cryptogenic stroke, it is evident the great majority are some form of embolism, not in situ occlusive disease of the brain arteries.

Lacunar Infarction

This set of syndromes is usually explained by infarction confined to the territory of a single small artery. In earlier years they were understood to be caused by a special arterial disease caused by hypertension. Only a small number of cases have had the underlying pathology proven. Because small infarcts are now commonly seen on CT or MR, the subject has become of much greater interest than it was when it was first proposed [18].

The risk factors for lacunar syndromes are the same as those for atherosclerosis of large arteries, and hypertension is no longer as crucial an issue as it was [19]. CT scanning is positive for roughly half of lacunar syndromes. MR has increased the yield somewhat. Although some cases of the pure motor stroke syndrome have been found associated with middle cerebral artery stenosis, this finding is uncommon, even rare, and pure motor stroke should not be thought of as a syndrome of large artery disease [20, 21]. The prognosis for reccurrence seems lower than that for other forms of brain infarction, suggesting there is a justifiable subset known as lacunes [22].

Infarct with Tandem Arterial Pathology

This category is uncommon but was thought for a time to be an important cause of stroke which would explain away the high frequency of cryptogenic cases. It has not. These are the cases of embolism from a carotid or vertebral source. They are known to occur but seem quite uncommon. The biggest risk factor for recurrence from carotid disease has been the degree of stenosis, not the presence of ulcerations alone.

Comparisons in the NINDS Stroke Data Bank (fig. 1, 2) between the 246 cardioembolic and 66 arterial embolic patients with cerebral infarction showed that, when controlled for differences in the frequency of cardiac disease, transient ischemic attacks and carotid bruits, artery-to-artery embolism was more frequent when a solitary superficial infarct was found by brain imaging or when the hematocrit was high [23]. By comparison, cardiac embolism was more frequent when the syndrome was large, as suggested by an impaired consciousness in the acute stage or by abnormal first CT. Thus, the location and extent of the cortical infarction differ somewhat in the two sources of emboli.

Infarct with Large Artery Thrombosis

Thrombosis of large arteries is now recognized to account for a small percentage of ischemic strokes. Even in the presence of large artery atherosclerosis, sufficient to cause hemodynamic stenosis, embolism clinically indistinguishable from that of cardiac origin, can occur from the lesion [24].

Stroke attributed to perfusion failure in the brain distal to the site of severe stenosis or occlusion of a major vessel is an uncommon cause of stroke but continues to attract much attention because it seems likely it requires surgery for its relief. For the patient suffering perfusion failure, studies of the Stroke Data Bank comparing demographic, stroke risk factors, clinical and radiologic features were made comparing the 246 cardioembolic and 113 large vessel atherosclerotic cerebral infarcts. Data bank definitions ensured more transient ischemic attacks in atherosclerotic infarcts and more cardiac disease in cardioembolic infarcts, but the diagnosis was distinguished further. Patients with fractional arm weakness (shoulder different from the hand), hypertension, diabetes, and male gender occurred more frequently in atherosclerotic than cardioembolic infarcts [25]. Atherosclerotic infarcts were more likely to have a fractional arm weakness regardless of infarct size. For the fractional weakness profile, it was inferred the high convexity, distal field location of the lesion accounted for such subtle signs compared with the larger, more proximally situated infarcts found in conventional embolism.

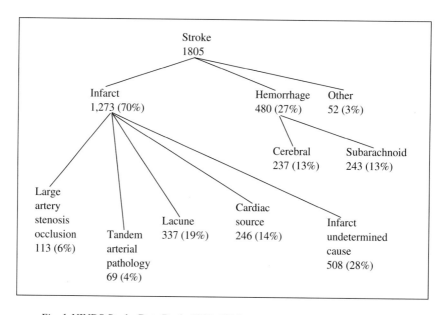

Fig. 1. NINDS Stroke Data Bank, 1983–1986.

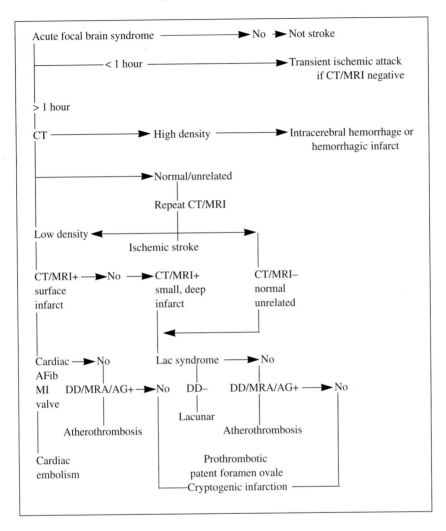

Fig. 2. Stroke diagnostic algorithm. DD = Duplex and transcranial Doppler; MRA = magnetic resonance angiography; AG = cerebral angiogram; CT = computerized tomography; MRI = magnetic resonance imaging. LAC syndrome refers to currently described classic lacunar syndromes, but may include other syndromes from focal-deep infarction (i. e. cognitive changes from thalamic or caudate infarcts).

The abnormalities on CT or MR scan or on PET scanning [26] reflecting the 'distal field' effect occur high over the convexity along the border zone between middle and anterior cerebral territories, especially on the middle cerebral side. The centripetal spread in more severe cases may involve so much of the hemisphere that a differentiation from embolism to the middle cerebral artery stem is impossible. Occlusions involving the territories of the anterior, middle, or posterior cerebral, or basilar artery territory are not distinguishable by brain image between thrombosis and embolism if the scan shows low density only in the proximal fields of the arterial territory. In all cases, any high-density component that suggests hemorrhagic infarction would favor a diagnosis of embolism.

Embolism Attributed to Cardiac or Transcardiac Source

Embolism of cardiac origin accounts for between 15 and 30% of cases, but when all forms of embolism are added up, they are the major cause of stroke explaining almost 50% of infarct cases. Most of them occur in the territory of the middle cerebral artery.

Embolic material is notoriously unstable, often disappearing within minutes to hours after the original occlusion. The persistence of embolic occlusion seems to be the exception rather than the rule. No reliable means have been developed to predict which type or size of embolic occlusions will persist and which will disappear. Embolic obstruction of an arterial lumen is cleared most commonly by recanalization and fibrinolysis [27]. Surprisingly, anterograde thrombus does not regularly develop through length of the vessel. This lack implies either an active flow proximal to the occlusion or that the occlusion was too short-lived to permit the development of an anterograde thrombus.

The many syndromes once considered specific for embolism have almost all fallen by the wayside: pure Wernicke's aphasia, isolated hemianopia, and monopareses. In the Lausanne Stroke Registry, hemianopia without hemiparesis or hemisensory disturbances, Wernicke's aphasia, ideomotor apraxia, involvement of specific territories (posterior division of middle cerebral artery, anterior cerebral artery, cerebellum, multiple territories), were associated with the presence of a potential cardiac source of embolism [28]. Further, the sudden onset once thought to typify embolism and the nonsudden onset thought typical of thrombosis are now well known to occur in either condition. Nonsudden or fluctuating onset occurs in 5–6%

of documented embolic strokes. The one syndrome which has held its value is the spectacular shrinking deficit, which can occur when the embolus is introduced into the internal carotid, causing a profound full hemisphere syndrome, after which it passes up the internal carotid to its final resting place in, say, the angular branch of the middle cerebral artery leaving only a mild aphasia after a few days or a week. Especially characteristic of the middle cerebral artery migratory embolism is the syndrome of fading hemiparesis with Wernicke's aphasia: the embolus lodges initially at the stem of the middle cerebral, occluding the penetrating lenticulostriate branches long enough to produce scattered foci of infarction through the basal ganglia and internal capsule, the involvement of the latter producing the hemiparesis. Distal migration of the embolus then occurs, finally occluding the lower division of the middle cerebral artery at the superior temporal plane and beyond. This infarct yields the Wernicke's aphasia. Two separate foci of infarction occur, but both result from the same embolic event.

In the Stroke Data Bank, besides a greater frequency of cardiac disease, patients with cardioembolic infarction more often presented with reduced consciousness [29]. Cardioembolic infarcts were more likely to have nonfractional arm weakness, except for those with infarctions less than 20 cm^3 where fractional weakness was more frequent. In a separate Stroke Data Bank analysis, history of systemic embolism and an abrupt onset were historical features significantly associated with cardiac sources of embolism. Clinical features observed at stroke onset help distinguish the cardioembolic group from other subtypes, but the diagnosis largely depends on confirmatory laboratory findings suggesting a definite cardiac source of embolism.

Zusammenfassung

Klassifikation von Schlaganfällen: Erfahrungen mit
Schlaganfalldateien

Fortschritte in der Technologie bildgebender Verfahren, wie CCT, NMR, Duplex, transkranieller Doppler und SPECT, haben die Möglichkeiten, einen verläßlichen Algorithmus für die Schlaganfalldiagnose zu erstellen, erheblich verbessert. Klinische Eindrücke können jetzt durch technische Daten erhärtet und Schlaganfalluntertypen unterschieden werden. Große Datenbanken können zudem bei der Aufdeckung von Risikofaktoren [Stroke 1991; 22:1491–1496], bei der Bestimmung des Stellenwertes bildgebender Verfahren [Stroke

1992;23:142], bei der Entdeckung seltener Schlaganfallformen, bei der Aufdeckung pathophysiologischer Mechanismen [Circulation 1991;83:172–175], bei der Validierung von Diagnose und Prognose, bei interinstitutionellen Vergleichen und bei der Vorbereitung klinischer Untersuchungen [Neurology 1991;41:33] nützlich sein.

Probleme der klinischen und der technischen Diagnose von Hirnblutungen: Die Diagnose von Blutungen ist durch CCT und NMR unproblematisch; Überlebenschancen hängen von Lokalisation und Größe ab [Ann Neurol 1989;26:131]. Gute NMR-Bilder erlauben die Diagnose von Kavernomen und kleinen arteriovenösen Fehlbildungen. Beide zeigen meist einen hyperintensen Fokus, der von einem hypointensen Ring umgeben ist. Eine Differenzierung von ischämischen Insulten und Blutungen ist aufgrund klinischer Daten allein nicht zuverlässig. Dies gilt insbesondere für kleine umschriebene Blutungen, bei denen Bewußtseinsstörungen, Kopfschmerz, Übelkeit und Erbrechen fehlen. Eine Abgrenzung von hämorrhagischen Infarzierungen ist allerdings ausschließlich aufgrund bildgebender Verfahren schwierig.

Probleme der klinischen und der technischen Diagnose von Infarkten: Die Algorithmen für die Klassifikation von Schlaganfalluntertypen sind erheblich verbessert worden, sind jedoch noch immer nicht zufriedenstellend. Aufgrund der großen Datensammlung der Stroke Data Bank ist eine Klassifikation nach angenommenen Schlaganfallmechanismen versucht worden. Diese Bemühungen haben einige Veränderungen bei den großen Infarktkategorien zur Folge gehabt. So wurde die Gruppe der atherothrombotischen Infarkte in zwei Untergruppen aufgeteilt: Infarkt aufgrund einer Thrombose eines großen Gefäßes und Infarkt durch arterio-arterielle Embolie. Trotz dieser Bemühungen verbleibt ein enttäuschend hoher Prozentsatz ungeklärter Schlaganfallursachen. Eine separate Kategorie – «Infarkt ungeklärter Genese» – hilft daher, die Homogenität der diagnostischen Gruppen der Stroke Data Bank zu sichern.

Infarkte ungeklärter Genese: Gründe für die ungenügende Klärung von Infarktursachen liegen darin, daß eine Abklärung nicht oder zu spät unternommen wurde und daher schon aufgelöste Emboli mittels Angiographie oder Doppler-Sonographie nicht mehr erfaßbar waren. Insgesamt machen Infarkte ungeklärter Genese etwa 40% aller Fälle aus. Ein kleiner Teil von ihnen kann durch hämatologische Erkrankungen, wie Protein-C- oder Protein-S-Mangel, Lupus-Antikoagulant oder Antikardiolipin-Antikörper, verursacht sein. Andere mögliche Ursachen sind paradoxe Embolien bei offenem Foramen ovale [Neurology 1992;42:16], selten Arteriitiden und Vasospasmen, wie sie z. B. bei der Migräne angenommen werden. Faßt man alle möglichen Ursachen der Infarkte ungeklärter Genese zusammen, so ergeben sich Hinweise darauf, daß die meisten von ihnen embolisch bedingt sein dürften.

Lakunen: Lakunen sind Infarkte im Versorgungsgebiet einzelner kleiner Arterien. Risikofaktoren für lakunäre Syndrome sind die gleichen wie für die Arteriosklerose der großen Gefäße [Stroke 1991;22:175–182]. Die CCT ist in etwa der Hälfte der Fälle lakunärer Syndrome positiv, die NMR etwas häufiger. Obwohl einige Patienten mit pure motor stroke Mediastenosen hatten, sollte dieses Syndrom nicht mit Makroangiopathie assoziiert werden. Die Rezidivrate lakunärer Insulte scheint geringer zu sein als die von anderen Hirninfarkten [Stroke 1987;18:545–551].

Infarkte bei arterieller Tandemläsion: Darunter versteht man die seltenen Fälle mit Embolien von Karotis oder Vertebralarterie. Vergleicht man in der NINDS Stroke Data Bank die 246 kardio-embolischen mit den 66 arterio-arteriellen Infarktpatienten, so zeigt sich, daß arterio-arterielle Embolien häufiger bei singulären superfiziellen Infarkten und bei hohem Hämatokrit zu finden waren [Neurology 1990;40(suppl 1):417]. Kardiale Embolien waren bei schweren Syndromen und bei abnormem Erst-CCT häufiger.

Infarkte bei Thrombose großer Arterien: Dieser Mechanismus verursacht nur einen kleinen Prozentsatz aller Infarkte. Selbst eine hochgradige Arterienstenose schließt aber eine embolische Genese des Schlaganfalles nicht aus. In einem Vergleich von 246 kardio-embolischen Infarkten mit 113 Infarkten aufgrund von Arteriosklerose großer Gefäße waren transitorische ischämische Attacken bei Patienten mit arteriosklerotischen und kardiale Erkrankungen bei kardio-embolischen Infarkten häufiger. Patienten mit partieller Armschwäche (Schulter anders als Hand), Hypertonie, Diabetes mellitus und männlichem Geschlecht waren bei arteriosklerotischen Infarkten häufiger als bei kardio-embolischen Infarkten [J Neurol 1990;237:140]. Pathologische Veränderungen in CCT, NMR oder PET finden sich entlang der Grenzzone zwischen vorderer und mittlerer Hirnarterie. Die Infarktausdehnung kann aber auch zentripetal so weit zur Media reichen, daß eine Unterscheidung von einem embolischen Insult nicht mehr möglich ist. Eine hämorrhagische Komponente spricht allerdings für Embolie.

Embolie kardialer oder transkardialer Ursache: Derartige Embolien machen 15–30% aller Hirninfarkte aus. Zählt man jedoch alle Formen der Embolie hinzu, kommt man auf fast 50% aller Fälle. Die meisten Embolien ereignen sich in der mittleren Hirnarterie. Embolisches Material ist instabil und verschwindet oft rasch. Prädiktoren für Persistenz oder Auflösung sind nicht bekannt. Anterograde Thrombosen kommen nach embolischen Verschlüssen nicht regelmäßig vor. Früher für embolische Infarkte als spezifisch angesehene Syndrome haben sich für die Beurteilung nicht als zuverlässig erwiesen. Selbst aufgrund eines plötzlichen oder eines verzögerten Beginns kann nicht ausreichend zwischen Embolie und Thrombose differenziert werden. Nur das rasch kleiner werdende Defizit (z. B. Beginn mit komplettem Hemisphärensyndrom, Rückbildung bis auf kortikales Defizit, wie Wernicke-Aphasie), ist für einen wandernden Embolus typisch. Insgesamt weisen kardio-embolische Insulte häufiger initiale Bewußtseinsstörungen, nichtpartielle Armlähmungen, abrupten Beginn und eine Vorgeschichte mit systemischen Embolien auf [Neurology 1990;40:281–284].

References

1   Sacco RL, Hauser WA, Mohr JP: Hospitalized stroke in Blacks and Hispanics in northern Manhattan. Stroke 1991;22:1491–1496.

2   Mohr JP, Biller J, Hilal SK, Yuh WTC, Chang DN, Tatemichi TK, Tali E, Nguyen H, Mun I, Adams HP Jr, Grisman K, Marler JR: MR vs. CT imaging in acute stroke. Stroke 1992;23:142.

3   Mohr JP: Natural history and pathophysiology of cerebral vascular disease. Circulation 1991;83:172–175.

4   Libman RB, Sacco RL, Shi T, Mohr JP: Spontaneous improvement in pure motor stroke: Implications for clinical trials. Neurology 1991;41:33.

5   Gorelick PB, Foulkes MA, Hier DB, Das A, Wolf P, Price T, Mohr JP: Predictors of ambulation following ischemic stroke: The Stroke Data Bank. Neurology 1992: 42(part 2):19.

6   Tatemichi TK, Foulkes MA, Mohr JP, Hewitt JR, Hier DB, Price TR, Wolf PA: Dementia in stroke survivors in the Stroke Data Bank cohort: Prevalence, incidence, risk factors, and computed tomographic findings. Stroke 1990;21:858–867.

7   Hier DB, Foulkes MA, Swiontoniowski M, Sacco RL, Gorelick PB, Mohr JP, Price TR,
     Wolf PA: Stroke recurrence within 2 years after ischemic infarction. Stroke
     1991;22:155–161.

8   Sacco RL, Foulkes MA, Mohr JP, Wolf PA, Hier DB, Price TR: Determinants of early
     recurrence of cerebral infarction. The Stroke Data Bank. Stroke 1989;20:983–989.

9   Melski JW, Caplan LR, Mohr JP, Geer DE, Bleich HL: Modeling the diagnosis of
     stroke at two hospitals. MD Comput 1989;6:157–163.

10   Tuhrim S, Dambrosia JM, Price TR, Mohr JP, Wolf PA, Hier DB, Kase CS: Intra-
     cerebral hemorrhage: Cross-validation and extension of a model for predicting 30-day
     survival. Ann Neurol 1989;26:131.

11   Massaro AR, Sacco RL, Mohr JP, Foulkes MA, Tatemichi TK, Wolf PA, Hier DB,
     Price TR: Clinical discriminators separate lobar and subcortical hemorrhage: The
     Stroke Data Bank. Neurology 1991;41:1881–1885.

12   Massaro AR, Sacco RL, Timsit SG, Mohr JP, Foulkes MA, Tatemichi TK, Hier DB,
     Price TR, Wolf PA: Early clinical discriminators between cerebral infarction and
     hemorrhagic stroke. Ann Neurol 1991;30:246–247.

13   Beghi E, Bogliun G, Cavaletti G, Sanguineti I, Tagliabue M, Agostoni F, Macchi I:
     Hemorrhagic infarction: Risk factors, clinical and tomographic features, and outcome.
     A case-control study. Acta Neurol Scand 1989;80:226–231.

14   Pessin MS, Hinton RC, Davis KR, Duncan GW, Mohr JP: Mechanisms of acute carotid
     stroke: A clinicoangiographic study. Ann Neurol 1979;6:245.

15   Mayer SA, Sacco RL, Hurlett-Jensen A, Shi T, Mohr JP: Free protein S deficiency and
     acute ischemic stroke. Stroke 1992;23:158.

16   Hart RG, Kanter MC: Hematologic disorders and ischemic stroke. A selective review.
     Stroke 1990;21:1111–1121.

17   DiTullio MR, Sacco RL, Homma S, Mohr JP: Variables associated with patent foramen
     ovale in young patients with stroke. Neurology 1992;42:157; Neurology 1992;42(part 2):16.

18   Hommel M, Besson G, Le Bas JF, Gaio JM, Pollak P, Borgel F, Perret J: Prospective
     study of lacunar infarction using magnetic resonance imaging. Stroke
     1990;21:546–554.

19   Chamorro AM, Sacco RL, Mohr JP, Foulkes MA, Kase CS, Tatemichi TK, Wolf PA,
     Price TR, Hier DB: Lacunar infarction: Clinical-CT correlations in the Stroke Data
     Bank. Stroke 1991;22:175–182.

20   Araki G: Small infarctions of the basal ganglia with special reference to transient
     ischemic attacks. Recent Adv Gerontol 1978;469:161.

21   Hinton RC, Mohr JP, Ackerman RA, Adair LB, Fisher CM: Symptomatic middle
     cerebral artery stem stenosis. Ann Neurol 1979;5:152.

22   Bamford J, Sandercock P, Jones L, Warlow C: The natural history of lacunar infarction:
     The Oxfordshire Community Stroke Project. Stroke 1987;18:545–551.

23   Timsit S, Sacco RL, Mohr JP, Foulkes MA, Tatemichi TK, Price TR, Hier DB, Wolf
     PA: Brain infarction severity differs according to cardiac or arterial embolic source:
     The NINDS Stroke Data Bank. Neurology 1990;40(suppl 1):417.

24   Castaigne, P, Lhermitte F, Gautier JC, et al: Arterial occlusions in the vertebro-basilar
     system – A study of forty-four patients with post-mortem data. Brain 1973;96:133.

25   Timsit S, Sacco RL, Mohr JP, Foulkes MA, Tatemichi TK, Wolf PA, Price TR, Hier
     DB: Early clinical differentiation of atherosclerotic and cardioembolic infarction:
     Stroke Data Bank. J Neurol 1990;237:140.

26 Baron JC, Frackowiak RS, Herholz K, Jones T, Lammertsma AA, Mazoyer B, Wienhard K: Use of PET methods for measurement of cerebral energy metabolism and hemodynamics in cerebrovascular disease. J Cereb Blood Flow Metab 1989;9:723–742.

27 Tohgi H, Kawashima M, Tamura K, Suzuki H: Coagulation fibrinolysis abnormalities in acute and chronic phases of cerebral thrombosis and embolism. Stroke 1990;21:1663–1667.

28 Bogousslavsky J, Cachin C, Regli F, Despland PA, Van-Melle G, Kappenberger L: Cardiac sources of embolism and cerebral infarction – clinical consequences and vascular concomitants: The Lausanne Stroke Registry. Neurology 1991;41:855–859.

29 Kittner SJ, Sharkness CM, Price TR, Plotnick GD, Dambrosia JM, Wolf PA, Mohr JP, Hier DB, Kase CS, Tuhrim S: Infarcts with a cardiac source of embolism in the NINDS Stroke Data Bank: Historical features. Neurology 1990;40:281–284.

Prof. J. P. Mohr, MD
Neurological Institute
Columbia University
710 West 168th Street
New York, NY 10032 (USA)

Dorndorf W, Marx P (eds): Stroke Prevention.
Basel, Karger, 1994, pp 14–27

Etiological Classification of Ischemic Strokes: Evidence from CT and SPECT Imaging[1]

E. B. Ringelstein[a], C. Weiller[b]

[a] Department of Neurology, Zentralklinikum ,WWU, University Hospital, Münster;
[b] Department of Neurology, University Hospital, Essen, FRG

We have elsewhere proposed a pathophysiologically oriented classification system for hemispheric brain infarctions visible on computerized tomography (CT) scans (fig. 1). Lesions indicating (1) cerebral microangiopathy (i. e. lacunes and subcortical arteriosclerotic encephalopathy), (2) low-flow infarctions within the terminal supply areas of the long penetrating arteries, or watershed infarctions of the frontolateral and temporoparieto-occipital cortex, and (3) territorial infarctions with damage of the major and minor pial artery territories were differentiated [1, 2]. The latter include a subcortical type of infarction, the so-called large striatocapsular infarct (LSCI) [1–4], which is also thought to be caused by a thromboembolic stroke mechanism.

In order to validate this classification system, several investigations had been performed during the last years. The questions addressed during these studies were: (1) What type of infarctions is seen in patients with proven embolic mechanism of stroke? (2) When does the subcortial type of territorial infarction, the so-called LSCI occur, and how can the concomitant cortical symptoms be explained? (3) Under which circumstances do internal carotid artery (ICA) occlusions lead to low-flow infarcts, thromboembolic infarcts or no infarcts at all?

[1] Parts of these investigations have been supported by the Alexander von Humboldt Foundation, Bonn-Godesberg, FRG.

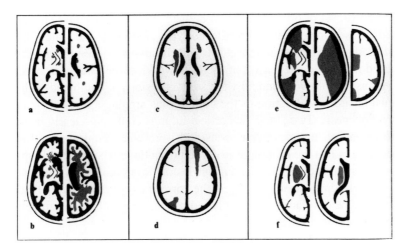

Fig. 1. Schematic drawing of pathogenetically different ischemic brain lesions. *a* Lacunar infarctions of typical site and size. Note multiplicity of lesions. *b* Subcortical arteriosclerotic encephalopathy (Binswanger's type) with multiple lacunae combined with diffuse periventricular white matter lesions and brain shrinkage. *c* Terminal supply area ('letzte Wiese') infarctions, the subcortical low-flow type of infarcts. The small periventricular lesion on the right is not clearly distinguishable from a single lacune. *d* Watershed infarctions between the main arterial territories involving cortex and subcortex. *e* Territorial infarctions of various sizes within the middle cerebral, anterior cerebral, and posterior cerebral artery territories. *f* Subcortical type of territorial infarction. The so-called 'large ganglionic infarction', i. e. LSCI or 'large lentiform nucleus infarction'. Note that the territory of the lenticulostriate arteries is infarcted in both its lower gray matter and upper white matter part [from 1].

Hemispheric Infarction due to Cardiogenic Embolism

In a previous study [5], 60 patients had been collected consecutively who fulfilled the following criteria: (1) Normal ultrasound findings of the extracranial brain arteries by means of continuous wave (CW) Doppler sonography; (2) normal findings during transcranial Doppler sonography (TCD) of the large intracranial arteries except for occlusions of the pial arteries directly involved; (3) a hemispheric infarction visible on CT and corresponding to the clinical deficit; (4) CT performed within 5 days at the latest after stroke onset, and (5) proven (n = 42) or clinically evident (n = 13) source of embolism within the heart. (6) Five additional patients had suffered a stroke due to catheter-related embolism.

In 55 (92%) of 60 patients, infarctions visible on CT could clearly be identified as belonging to the territorial type. Lesions of the watershed or terminal supply area type were not found. Infarctions resembling lacunes occurred in 5 cases. At least 2 of them, however, turned out to be wedge-shaped instead of ovoid and all were solitary lesions or combined with additional territorial infarction of the cortex, thus arguing against their lacunar pathogenesis. Two small subcortical infarcts could not clearly be attributed to one of the above categories and were considered unclassifiable. Seven lesions met the criteria of LSCI, representing the subcortical type of territorial infarcts (see below). Multiple lesions were seen in 11 patients.

These findings strongly suggest the correctness of our concept that the territorial type of infarction is highly indicative of an embolic origin, either cardiac or arterio-arterial in genesis.

Occurrence of LSCI and Their Relation to Cortical Deficits

In a recent study [6], we evaluated the influence of time of recanalization of the middle cerebral artery (MCA) or degree of initial leptomeningeal collateral blood flow within the first 6 h after stroke onset in cardioembolic or arterio-arterial MCA occlusions on infarct size and clinical outcome in a series of 34 consecutive acute stroke patients. They had either occlusion of the mainstem (n = 31) or major branch (n = 3) of the MCA. Patients were investigated by means of CT, very early cerebral arteriography (n = 21; < 6 h), and repetitive close-meshed TCD. By means of TCD, the time span was defined within which recanalization must have occurred. This period began with the time of the last TCD study when the MCA was still occluded, and ended with the first reappearance of a flow signal within this artery. Accordingly, patients were arbitrarily subdivided into 3 groups with 'very early' (< 4 h), 'early' (> 4–8 h), or 'late' (> 8 h) MCA recanalization. The size of the definite final infarct on CT was assessed within 2 weeks after stroke. The type and size of infarction was related to the initial arteriographic findings, in particular to the quality of the leptomeningeal collateral blood flow. The degree of leptomeningeal collateralization on the initial arteriogram was roughly quantified as good, moderate or poor according to the number of major MCA branches showing retrograde filling during the early venous phase. Twenty-two patients (65%) showed recanalization of their occluded MCAs within 3 days. This proportion rose to 26 (76%) within the entire 17-day observation period.

Only a synoptic comparison of the time of recanalization and the extent of leptomeningeal collateralization with the infarct size or clinical outcome revealed findings in the expected direction. Subgroups of patients who had a good/moderate leptomeningeal collateralization *and* an MCA recanalization within 4 or 8 h, most often presented with relatively small infarcts, particularly the prognostically relatively benign, purely subcortical LSCI, as opposed to those with poor leptomeningeal network and later recanalization. The difference in infarct size was statistically significant. Even highly significant differences were found if these parameters were related to the clinical outcome.

Depending on the site of occlusion within the MCA, the size and the topographic distribution of ensuing lesions varied considerably but shared certain uniform features within each subgroup (fig. 2). With only 1 exception, patients with a proximal MCA occlusion (n = 18/21) always developed ischemic damage at least in the territory of the deep perforators. In 5 of them (24%), the LSCI was seen without cortical involvement on CT. More distally located emboli/thromboses (n = 3/21) spared the lenticulostriate territory and led to infarctions of the white matter and cortex.

These findings indicate that analysis of the location and extension of the infarct on CT allows the reconstruction, to some degree, of the initial location of the MCA occlusion. Obviously, infarction of the basal ganglia is unavoidable in proximal MCA occlusion blocking the orifices of the deep perforators. This confirms that the lenticulostriate vessels are end-arteries with no possibility of anastomotic collateral blood flow. In accordance with similar findings published recently [7, 8], the presence of a collateral leptomeningeal circulation reduces infarct size and improves clinical outcome. The presence of a good collateral blood supply, however, does not reliably limit the extension of the infarct in every case and seems to constitute only one of several important factors in the natural history of embolic MCA occlusions. We hypothesize that the extent of the leptomeningeal blood supply defines the temporal width of the therapeutic window.

In another study [4], we examined 29 patients with strictly subcortical LSCI by means of TCD or intra-arterial selective arteriography, CT scanning and single ^{99m}Tc-hexamethyl-propylenamine oxime-single photon emission computed tomography (HMPAO-SPECT) within 4 weeks after stroke onset. SPECT was used to assess cerebral blood flow, blood volume, and cerebral perfusion reserve. Eight of the patients had aphasia or neglect, the residual 21 cases did not show any cortical deficits. On both

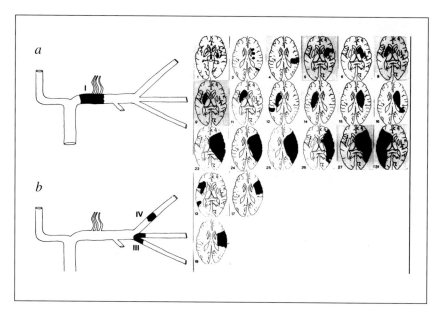

Fig. 2. Relation between localization of the occluding process within the MCA axis and the type and size of infarction visible on CT. *a* In proximal MCA occlusions (n = 18; I), the thrombus or embolus always blocked the mouths of the long perforators leading to infarction of the basal ganglia. Two exceptions (panels 2, 4) can be explained by very rapid MCA recanalization. Depending on leptomeningeal collateral blood flow or rapidity of recanalization, or both, the cortex may remain more or less intact (see panels 1, 5, 6, 8, 9, 11, 12, 14, 15, 16). *b* In isolated (IV) or dual (III) MCA branch occlusions (n = 3) (panels 13, 17, 19), infarctions are restricted mainly to the corresponding vascular territory of the cortex leaving the basal ganglia intact [from 6].

CT scans and magnetic resonance imaging, the infarcts corresponded exactly to the territories of the medial and lateral group of the lenticulostriate arteries, Heubner's artery, or the anterior choroidal artery. The infarctions had occurred either due to cerebral embolization into the M1 segment of the MCA or due to stenoses at the same site. In any case, these large vessel lesions had acutely and simultaneously occluded the orifices of the lenticulostriate or neighboring arteries.

A persistent occlusion of the MCA and a decrease of cortical regional cerebral blood flow (rCBF) were only found in patients with aphasia or neglect, whereas all patients without cortical deficits showed a rapid re-

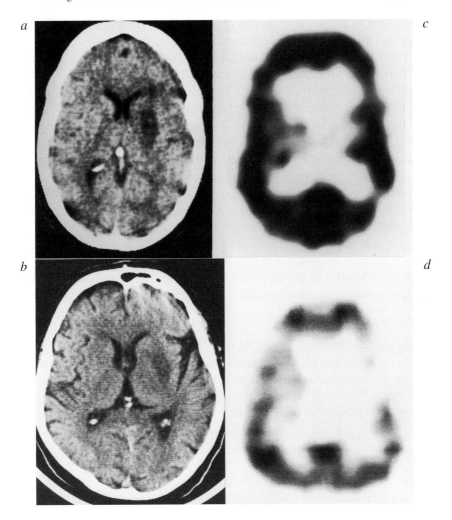

Fig. 3. Comparison of a corresponding rCBF and CT slice in a patient with and without aphasia. *a* LSCI on the left. *b* The rCBF decrease is confined to the region of interest corresponding to the subcortical infarcted area seen in figure 3a. The stroke was caused by cardiac embolization from a mural thrombus. *c* Similar LSCI in another patient with aphasia. Again, the infarcted area on CT is restricted to the striatocapsular distribution on the left. *d* The rCBF, however, is decreased in the subcortical infarcted area, as well as in large parts of the cortical MCA territory [modified from 4].

canalization of the MCA occlusion or a stenosis of the M1 segment of the MCA, and no cortical rCBF decrease (fig. 3).

From these findings we concluded that the neuropsychological deficits in patients with LSCI can be explained by decreased cortical blood flow due to a persistent or long-lasting occlusive lesion of the MCA in the absence of sufficient leptomeningeal collaterals. While some authors attribute these cortical symptoms to basal ganglia participation in the processing of speech [11], these deficits can also be explained by solely functional involvement of the cortex itself (= diaschisis), i. e. transient depression of function occurring at a distance from a focal cerebral lesion [12]. By contrary, we support the hypothesis that the cortical deficit is caused by a selective ischemic neuron disease (so-called 'elektive Parenchymnekrose' according to Spatz [9]), which had been shown microscopically in two comparable cases by Lassen et al. [10]. In LSCI, a decreased cortical rCBF, if present, is caused by a critically reduced perfusion pressure due to a persistent occlusive lesion of the MCA. The decreased cortical rCBF yields to a decreased cortical metabolism and to cortical symptoms such as aphasia or neglect. Rapid recanalization of the occluded MCA and excellent leptomeningeal collateral blood flow may prevent patients from having cortical deficits.

Because of the clinical features, the rCBF pattern, and the pathogenetic mechanisms described, LSCI belong to the territorial type of infarct caused by large vessel disease. Terms like super lacune or giant lacune [11] should be avoided since they imply a completely different pathogenesis, i. e. small vessel disease, and may lead to inadequate diagnostic and therapeutic decisions.

The Key Role of the Circle of Willis for the Pathogenesis of Low-Flow Infarctions

PET studies in patients with severe occlusive disease of the ICA have shown that areas of diminished or even paradoxical CO_2 reactivity correspond precisely to areas of compensatory vasodilation which counterbalances the reduced perfusion pressure [13], and that such areas exactly coincide with a critical, upper limit oxygen extraction rate [14]. Thus, it was expected that cerebral vasomotor reactivity (VMR) would be greatly reduced in patients with low-flow infarctions on CT, but much less so in patients with the thromboembolic type of brain lesions. It was further hypothesized that the collateral capacity of the circle of Willis was the major determinant of the hemodynamic impact of severe extracranial occlusive disease.

Sixty-five consecutive patients with unilateral or bilateral ICA occlusions were selected, 19 had been asymptomatic and 46 had suffered transient ischemic attacks (n = 9) or completed strokes or both. A CT scan was obtained in each patient at least once within a week after the last ischemic event. Infarctions visible on CT were classified according to the system mentioned above. CO_2-induced VMR measurements were thought a suitable approach to determine the hemodynamic background of different types of brain infarctions by an independent test reflecting cerebral perfusion pressure. Details of the VMR measurement within the MCA territory are described elsewhere [15], and were performed between 6 weeks and 3 months after the acute ischemic event. In 45 patients, the cerebral collateral circulation using TCD during carotid compression could also be analyzed. From the flow phenomena at the intracranial large arteries during compression maneuvers at the ipsilateral (and contralateral) common carotid artery, one could infer the functional capacity of the circle of Willis (A = full collateralization via both the anterior and posterior communicating artery; B = exclusively anterior and C = exclusively posterior collateralization; D = 'isolated' MCA with blood supply only via a retrogradely irrigated ophthalmic artery.) It was hypothesized that a poorest collateral system would be associated with a lowest cerebral perfusion pressure, and, simultaneously, with an increased frequency of low-flow infarctions.

Twenty patients (subgroup 1) had no visible infarction on both initial and repeat CTs. While 28 patients (subgroup 2) showed infarction of the territorial, i. e. thromboembolic type, 16 cases (subgroup 3) revealed low-flow induced lesions. The most remarkable finding was that VMR was nearly identical in subgroup 1 with no infarctions (mean 48 ± 20) and subgroup 2 with thromboembolic, territorial-type infarctions (mean $49 \pm 20\%$), but both were significantly reduced as compared to normal values from a control group (mean VMR values $86 \pm 16\%$ [according to 15]). In subgroup 3, however, cerebral vasomotor reactivity was even more reduced (mean $28 \pm 22\%$). The differences between subgroups 1 and 3 or subgroups 2 and 3 were highly significant (p = 0.006 and 0.003; U test). The type and extent of collateralization via the circle of Willis or the ophthalmic artery revealed a relationship to the type of brain infarction on CT. While only 3 of 28 patients (11%) with cross-filling via the anterior collateral pathway of the circle of Willis (groups A and B) had low-flow infarctions, this proportion rose to 28% in patients with exclusively posterior cross-filling (group C), and even to 44% (4/9) if collateral blood flow to the depleted hemisphere relied on the ophthalmic artery alone (group D). The difference between groups A and B as compared to groups C and D was significant ($p < 0.05$). The decreasing collateralizing capacity of the circle of Willis correlated with reduction of VMR in the corresponding MCA territories. In ICA occlusions with anterior cross-filling, mean VMR values were 52 ± 16%. If hemispheric blood supply depended on the posterior communicating artery alone, VMR was slightly lower (45 ± 18%). However, in patients whose MCA blood supply was dependent on the ophthalmic artery, VMR was substantially lower (27 ± 21%). In other words, occlusions with and without good collateralization differed highly significantly in their vasoreactivity responses.

In conclusion, measurements of cerebral vasomotor reserve in patients with carotid-borne brain infarctions confirmed our hypothesis that in territorial thromboembolic infarcts this reserve is no less reduced than in patients with normal CTs but is dramatically diminished in low-flow infarctions. This supports the view that morphology of hemispheric infarctions on CT permits to retrospectively identify the underlying stroke mechanism in the majority of patients. This knowledge will help to choose the most adequate diagnostic and therapeutic strategies.

Shortcomings of the Classification System

There are certain weaknesses of the above typology of brain infarctions on CT predominantly due to equivocal appearance of various types of small subcortical infarctions. It is particularly difficult to differentiate 'solitary' lacunes from small 'striatocapsular infarcts' due to MCA-large vessel disease, and from small low-flow infarctions in the terminal supply area of the centrum semiovale [16, 17]. Solitary lesions with fuzzy edges in the subcortical white matter are rather terminal supply area infarctions than lacunes. The latter are multiple and preferably found in the striatum or capsule, sharply demarcated, ovoid in shape and small in size, whereas small variants of the LSCI are often triangular or wedge-shaped.

Another problematic issue are infarctions at the temporo-parieto-occipital junction of the cortex [18]. It is hardly possible to unequivocally differentiate between a posterior watershed infarction and a small territorial type of infarct in the most dorsal MCA distribution, unless additional low-flow infarcts are seen in the same hemisphere or cerebral VMR has been proven to be dramatically reduced.

Two questions are frequently raised by critical colleagues, namely (1) how could we explain that a patient with a typical low-flow infarct on CT may have a normal or only moderately reduced cerebrovascular reserve in the corresponding MCA distribution, and (2) how come that we occasionally see territorial types of infarctions in patients with ICA occlusions with a strongly reduced vasomotor reserve? We know from long-term follow-up studies [unpubl. data] that an initially exhausted cerebrovascular reserve, causing low-flow infarction, has a strong tendency to improve spontaneously over time within weeks and months, finally ending up with a 'nearly' normal cerebrovascular reserve. In the individual case, a strong reduction in vasomotor reserve strongly increases the probability of low-flow lesions but does not necessarily lead to them. An ICA occlusion being hemodynamically relevant does not prevent it to be, simultaneously, embolically active.

Conclusions

Our findings, supported by the recent reports of others [16, 19], indicate that low-flow hemispheric infarctions are associated with loss of CO_2-induced VMR. This supports the view that a long-lasting critical drop in perfusion pressure in the MCA territory is related to the occurrence of low-flow infarcts. Since VMR had turned out to be normal in patients with large hemispheric infarctions due to cardiac embolism [20], its reduction is not secondary to decreased tissue flow demands following stroke. The configuration of the circle of Willis is the most significant determinant of low-flow brain infarctions [19, 20]. Lack of sufficient collateral pathways for an anterior or posterior cross-filling is more frequently found in the low-flow group than in others. Retrograde flow via the ophthalmic artery indicates a severe intracranial hemodynamic insufficiency, since this pathway is only recruited as a collateral channel if both communicating arteries of the circle of Willis are unavailable or insufficient. Only a marginal collateral capacity is provided by the ophthalmic artery or other small ECA-fed vessels.

A territorial pattern of infarction, more or less identical to the described vascular distributions, may occur for two different reasons. In situ thrombosis may be superimposed on atherosclerotic plaques of the large intracranial cerebral arteries, or emboli from extracranial sources may block large pial arteries and their branches. The former represent only a minor subgroup of the stroke population [21–23]. Approximately half of the territorial infarctions are of arterioembolic origin from thrombotically active, ulcerated plaques, high-grade stenoses, or occlusions of the internal carotid arteries. Another considerable proportion of territorial infarcts is caused by cardiac emboli [5]. Thus, analysis of the type of infarction visible on CT may help to direct both the diagnostic workup of individual patients and future scientific studies towards the true pathogenesis of ischemic stroke.

Zusammenfassung

Ätiologische Klassifizierung von Hirninfarkten mit CCT und SPECT

Wir haben eine ätiologische Klassifizierung ischämischer Insulte der Großhirnhemisphären nach CCT-Kriterien vorgeschlagen [Fortschr Neurol Psychiatr 1985;53:315–36): 1. Läsionen, die für eine *Mikroangiopathie* indikativ sind, wie Lakunen und die arteriosklerotische Enzephalopathie; 2. *hämodynamisch bedingte Infarkte,* die sich entweder in der Endzone des Versorgungsareals der Aa. lenticulostriatae oder als Grenzzoneninfarkte manifestieren; 3. *Territorialinfarkte* in den Versorgungsgebieten größerer oder kleinerer pialer Arterien. Zur Validierung dieses Konzeptes sind mehrere Untersuchungen durchgeführt worden.

Hemisphäreninfarkte bei kardiogenen Embolien: In einer Untersuchung an 60 konsekutiven Patienten mit embolisch verursachten Großhirninfarkten [Ann Neurol 1989;26:759–765] zeigten 55 (92%) das Bild eines Territorialinfarktes. Grenz- oder Endzoneninfarkte fanden sich nicht. Fünf Infarkte ähnelten Lakunen, die jedoch alle solitär oder mit zusätzlichen Territorialinfarkten kombiniert waren. Zwei von ihnen boten statt des für Lakunen typischen ovoiden Aussehens ein trianguläres Bild; zwei weitere kleine subkortikale Läsionen konnten nicht eindeutig klassifiziert werden. Diese Befunde untermauern unsere Hypothese, daß Territorialinfarkte starke Indikatoren für kardiale oder arterio-arterielle Embolien sind.

Große striatokapsuläre Infarkte und ihre Beziehung zu kortikalen Defiziten: In einer Studie an 34 konsekutiven Patienten mit embolisch bedingten Hirninfarkten untersuchten wir den Einfluß der Rekanalisationszeit der Arteria cerebri media und des initialen leptomeningealen Kollateralkreislaufes auf Infarktgröße und klinisches Ergebnis. 31 Kranke hatten einen Verschluß des Mediahauptstammes, 3 einen größeren Astverschluß der Arteria cerebri media. Alle Patienten wurden mit CCT und wiederholten transkraniellen Doppler-Sonographien untersucht. 21 wurden innerhalb von 6 h angiographiert. 22 Patienten (65%) zeigten eine Rekanalisation innerhalb von 3 Tagen; nach 17 Tagen waren 26 (76%) rekanalisiert. Patienten mit relativ gutem leptomeningealem Kollateralfluß und/oder Rekanalisation innerhalb von 4 oder 8 h hatten meist nur kleine Infarkte, darunter die prognostisch relativ günstigen subkortikalen striatokapsulären Infarkte. Kranke mit schlechter Kollateralisation und später Rekanalisation hatten signifikant größere Infarkte und schlechtere klinische Befunde. Größe und topographische Ausdehnung hingen wesentlich vom Sitz des arteriellen Verschlusses ab. Proximale Mediahauptstammverschlüsse verursachten mit einer Ausnahme Infarkte im Versorgungsgebiet der striolentikulären Arterien. Bei 5 (24%) fand sich keine zusätzliche kortikale Beteiligung. Bei den 3 Patienten mit distalen Verschlüssen fanden sich Infarkte von weißer Substanz und Kortex ohne Beteiligung der Stammganglien. Diese Untersuchung zeigt, daß Infarktlokalisation und -größe Hinweise auf den Ort des Gefäßverschlusses zulassen. Bei proximalen Mediaverschlüssen mit Blockierung der striolentikulären Arterien sind Basalganglieninfarkte unvermeidbar. Eine gute kollaterale Versorgung kann oft, aber nicht immer, das Infarktausmaß verkleinern. Der Kollateralfluß kann das Spektrum der therapeutischen Maßnahmen bestimmen. In einer weiteren Studie [Arch Neurol 1990;47:1085–1091] haben wir 29 Patienten mit großen striatokapsulären Infarkten ohne erkennbare kortikale Begleitinfarkte im CCT oder NMR mit transkranieller Doppler-Sonographie oder früher Angiographie sowie HMPAO-SPECT innerhalb von 4 Wochen nach dem Infarkt untersucht. 8 dieser Patienten hatten kortikale Symptome, wie Aphasie oder Neglekt, die übrigen 21 nicht. Ein persistierender Verschluß der Arteria cerebri media und eine regionale kortikale Verminderung des zerebralen Blutflusses wurden nur bei Patienten mit kortikalen Symptomen gefunden. Kortikale Symptome bei Stammganglieninfarkten sind somit Ausdruck einer kortikalen Minderperfusion, und unsere Hypothese ist, daß sie einer elektiven Parenchymnekrose [Dtsch Z Nervenheilkd 1935;136:86–132] entsprechen.

Schlüsselrolle des Circulus arteriosus Willisii für die Pathogenese von hämodynamisch bedingten Infarkten: Zur Beantwortung dieser Frage wurden 65 Patienten mit ein- oder beidseitigem Internaverschluß ausgewählt. 19 waren asymptomatisch, 46 hatten transitorische ischämische Attacken oder Infarkte oder beides erlitten. Bei allen Patienten wurde während der 1. Woche nach dem letzten ischämischen Ereignis mindestens eine CCT durchgeführt. Die zerebrale vasomotorische Reaktivität (VMR) wurde nach 6 Wochen bis 3 Monaten mit dem CO_2-Test bestimmt [Stroke 1988;19:963–969]. Bei 45 Kranken konnte die zerebrale Kollateralzirkulation mit transkranieller Doppler-Sonographie analysiert werden. Die VMR betrug bei Kontrollen 86 ± 16, bei 20 Patienten ohne erkennbaren Hirninfarkt 48 ± 20, bei 28 Patienten mit Territorialinfarkt 49 ± 20 und bei 16 Patienten mit hämodynamisch verursachten Infarkten 28 ± 22%. Alle Gruppenunterschiede waren signifikant. Hämodynamisch bedingte Infarkte zeigten 3 von 28 Patienten (11%) mit Kollateralzufluß über den vorderen Anteil, 28% der Patienten mit ausschließlichem Zufluß über den hinteren Anteil des Circulus arteriosus Willisii und 4 von 9 Kranken (44%) mit ausschließlichem Zufluß über die Arteria ophthalmica. Die VMR war bei vorderer oder hinterer Kollateralisation mäßig (52 ± 16 bzw. 45 ± 18%), bei ausschließlichem Zufluß über die A. ophthalmica stärker (27 ± 21%) reduziert. Insgesamt zeigen diese Untersuchungen, daß hämodynamisch bedingte Infarkte bei Patienten auftreten, deren VMR stark (>3 SD) vermindert ist. Ein insuffizienter Circulus arteriosus Willisii ist der maßgebliche pathogenetische Faktor.

Probleme des Klassifikationssystems: Es ist sehr schwer, solitäre Lakunen von kleinen Endzoneninfarkten im Centrum semiovale und von kleinen striokapsulären Infarkten aufgrund von Makroangiopathien zu unterscheiden. Grenzzonen- und Territorialinfarkte im hinteren Mediastromgebiet sind, wenn zusätzliche Grenzzoneninfarkte fehlen, kaum zu differenzieren. Bei hämodynamisch bedingten Infarkten kann sich die VMR wieder normalisieren. Auch vollständige Verschlüsse der A. Carotis interna können embolisch Territorialinfarkte verursachen.

References

1 Ringelstein EB, Zeumer H, Schneider R: Der Beitrag der zerebralen Computertomographie zur Differentialtypologie und Differentialtherapie des ischämischen Großhirninfarktes. Fortschr Neurol Psychiatr 1985;53:315–336.

2 Ringelstein EB, Zeumer H, Angelou D: The pathogenesis of strokes from internal carotid artery occlusion. Diagnostic and therapeutical implications. Stroke 1983;14:867–875.

3 Bladin PF, Berkovics SF: Striatocapsular infarction: Large infarcts in the lenticulostriate arterial territory. Neurology 1984;34:1423–1430.

4 Weiller C, Ringelstein EB, Reiche W, Thron A, Buell U: The large striatocapsular infarct. A clinical and pathophysiological entity. Arch Neurol 1990;47:1085–1091.

5 Ringelstein EB, Koschorke S, Holling A, Thron A, Lambertz H, Minale C: Computed tomographic patterns of proven embolic brain infarctions. Ann Neurol 1989;26:759–765.

6 Ringelstein EB, Biniek R, Weiller C, Ammeling B, Nolte PN, Thron A: Type and extent of hemispheric brain infarctions and clinical outcome in early and delayed middle cerebral artery recanalization. Neurology 1992;42:289–298.

7 Saito I, Segawa H, Shiokawa Y, Taniguchi M, Tsutsumi K: Middle cerebral artery occlusion: Correlation of computed tomography and angiography with clinical outcome. Stroke 1987;18:863–868.

8 Bozzao L, Fantozzi LM, Bastinello S, Bozzao A, Fieschi C: Early collateral blood supply and late parenchymal brain damage in patients with middle cerebral artery occlusion. Stroke 1989;20:735–740.

9 Spatz H: Über die Beteiligung des Gehirns bei der von Winiwarter-Bürgerschen Krankheit (Thrombendangitis obliterans). Dtsch Z Nervenheilkd 1935;136:86–132.

10 Lassen NA, Olsen TS, Højgaard K, Skriver E: Incomplete infarction: A CT-negative irreversible ischemic brain lesion. J Cereb Blood Flow Metab 1983;3(suppl 1):602–603.

11 Crosson B, Novack TA, Trennery MR: Subcortical language mechanism: Window on a new frontier; in Whitacker HA (ed): Phonological Processes and Brain Mechanisms. New York, Springer, 1988; pp 25–29.

12 Baron JC, D'Antona RD, Pantano P, Serdaru M, Samson Y, Bousser MG: Effects of thalamic stroke on energy metabolism of the cerebral cortex. Brain 1986;109:1243–1259.

13 Levine RL, Sunderland JJ, Lagreze HL, Nickles RJ, Rose BR, Turski PA: Cerebral perfusion reserve indexes determined by fluoromethane positron emission scanning. Stroke 1988;19:19–27.

14 Kanno I, Uemura K, Higano S, Murakami M, Iieda H, Miura S, Shishido F, Inugami A, Sayama I: Oxygen extraction fraction at maximally vasodilated tissue in the ischemic brain estimated from the regional CO_2 responsiveness measured by positron emission tomography. J Cereb Blood Flow Metab 1988;8:227–235.

15 Ringelstein EB, Sievers C, Ecker S, Schneider PA, Otis SM: Noninvasive assessment of CO_2-induced cerebral vasomotor reactivity in normal individuals and patients with internal carotid artery occlusions. Stroke 1988;19:963–969.

16 Bogousslavsky J, Regli F: Unilateral watershed infarcts. Neurology 1986;36:373–377.

17 Leblanc R, Yamamoto YI, Taylor JL, Diksic M, Hakim A: Border zone ischemia. Ann Neurol 1987;22:707–713.

18   Gastaut H, Nagwet R, Vigorous RA: The vascular syndrome of the parietotemporo-occipital 'triangle' based on 18 cases; in Zülch KJ (ed): Cerebral Circulation and Stroke. Berlin, Springer, 1991, pp 82–92.

19   Keunen RWM, Ackerstaff RGA, Stegeman DF, Schulte BPM: The impact of internal carotid artery occlusion and of the integrity of the circle of Willis on cerebral vasomotor reactivity – A transcranial Doppler study; in Meyer JS, et al (eds): Cerebral Vascular Disease. Amsterdam, Elsevier Science Publishers, 1989, pp 85–88.

20   Weiller C, Ringelstein EB, Reiche W, Buell U: Clinical and hemodynamic aspects of low-flow infarcts. Stroke 1991;22:1117–1123.

21   Norrving B, Nielsson B, Risberg J: rCBF in patients with carotid occlusion: Resting and hypercapnic flow related to collateral patterns. Stroke 1982;13:155–162.

22   Bladin PF, Berkovic SF: Striatocapsular infarcts in the lenticulostriate arterial territory. Neurology 1984;34:1423–1430.

23   Santamaria J, Graus F, Rubio F, Abbizu T, Peres J: Cerebral infarction of the basal ganglia due to embolism from the heart. Stroke 1983;14:911–914.

Prof. Dr. E. B. Ringelstein
Klinik und Poliklinik für Neurologie
Zentralklinikum der WWU Münster
Albert-Schweitzer-Straße 33
D-48129 Münster (FRG)

Dorndorf W, Marx P (eds): Stroke Prevention.
Basel, Karger, 1994, pp 28–36

Cranial Computerized Tomography Stroke Patterns in Patients with Cardiac Sources of Embolism, Extracranial Macroangiopathy or No Extracranial Sources

H. Mast, F. Nüssel, H.P. Vogel, T. Heinsius, R. Dissmann, H. Völler, P. Marx

Abteilung Neurologie, Universitätsklinikum Steglitz der Freien Universität Berlin, BRD

The question of associations between cranial computerized tomography (CCT) patterns and stroke mechanisms like cardiac sources of embolism and extracranial macroangiopathy was addressed in a prospective study of 200 consecutive patients with ischemic stroke or transient ischemic attack (TIA). Doppler sonographic and echocardiographic (transthoracic and transesophageal) investigations were planned for each patient enrolled. CCT scan rating was done in a masked setting.

The null hypothesis of the study was an even distribution of CCT pattern frequencies among groups with different stroke mechanisms, the alternative hypothesis being a significant preponderance of pial-artery infarcts in patients with cardiac sources of embolism, low-flow infarcts in cases with carotid-artery stenoses, and lacunes in hypertensive individuals with no signs of macroangiopathy or cardiac sources of embolism.

Patients and Methods

The study included 200 unselected, consecutive patients presenting with an acute ischemic neurologic deficit to Steglitz Medical Center of the Free University of Berlin. The mean age, sex ratio, and risk factor profile are outlined in table 1. Those patients were labeled hypertensive who were on antihypertensive medications before the classifying event or who showed persistent blood pressure elevation (> 160/95 mm Hg), but not those with only tran-

Table 1. Baseline characteristics of 200 ischemic stroke patients

Characteristics	n	%
Age, mean (range): 58.5 (17–84)		
Sex, F/M	78/122	39/61
Risk factors – total	159	79.5
Subgroups[1]:		
Hypertension	92	46.0
Diabetes mellitus	43	21.5
Smoking	87	43.5
History of cardiac diseases – total	62	31
Subgroups[1]:		
Myocardial infarction	32	16
Coronary heart disease	20	10
Others[2]	20	10
Neurologic deficits		
Transient ischemic attack	39	19.5
Reversible ischemic deficit	58	29.0
Completed stroke	103	51.5

[1] Note that patients could have more than one risk factor and more than one cardiac disease which causes the sums of subgroups to exceed totals.
[2] Pacemaker (n = 9), valve operation (n = 1), myocardial insufficiency (n = 7), hypertrophic cardiomyopathy (n = 1), endocarditis (n = 1), operation of ventricular septum defect (n = 1).

sient rises during the initial stroke phase. Neurologic deficits were reversible in 97 (TIA 39, reversible ischemic neurological deficit 58 cases) and irreversible in 103 patients. In 33 patients the ischemic event occurred in the posterior circulation.

CCT scans were taken within the first week after stroke onset. The neuroradiologist (F.N.), who was masked with regard to clinical diagnoses and additional laboratory findings, classified the CCT images as follows: (1) pial-artery infarcts; (2) small deep infarcts (lacunes); (3) low-flow (border-zone) infarcts; (4) unclassified ischemic lesions, and (5) normal. Additionally, infarcts were rated as either fresh, old or age unknown. CCT pattern classification was done according to the proposed criteria of Mohr and Barnett [2], the Stroke Data Bank [6] and definitions set by Ringelstein et al. [1, 3]. Lacunes were defined as small (≤ 1.5 cm in diameter) deep infarcts in the vascular distribution of the striatolenticular arteries. Low-density lesions in the frontal and central suprasylvian region with sparing of the sylvian fissure and striatolenticular vessel areas were considered to be low-flow infarcts in the border zones of middle and anterior cerebral arteries. Low-flow infarcts were also assumed in band-like subcortical lesions in the distal lenticulostriate supply areas. Other lesions encompassing either cortical or subcortical as well as cortical structures and also hypodensities in the nucleus lentiformis with diameters of more than 1.5 cm were rated as pial-artery infarcts. Repeated CCT investigations were not mandatory.

Patients enrolled were investigated by extra- and transcranial Doppler sonography and B-scan as well as transthoracic and transesophageal echocardiography (ECHO). B-scan and transcranial Doppler sonography were not available for all cases included. All individuals had an electrocardiography (ECG). Sonographic and ECG results were to be used for assignment to one of three groups of stroke mechanisms:

(1) Cardiac source of embolism: (a) left ventricular or left atrial thrombus, no signs of macroangiopathy; (b) atrial fibrillation, no signs of macroangiopathy; (c) one or more of the following accepted sources of embolism [2]: mitral valve prolapse or calcification, prior myocardial infarction (within 6 weeks), possible transcardiac cause of stroke (septum defect, patent foramen ovale, right-to-left shunt), septum aneurysm, atrial myxoma, endocarditis (bacterial or marantic), wall-motility dysfunction; no signs of macroangiopathy.

(2) Macroangiopathy: carotid- or vertebral-artery stenosis.

(3) No cardiac source, no signs of macroangiopathy: (a) with hypertension or (b) without hypertension.

Given the expected high coincidence of extracranial arterial stenoses and cardiac sources of embolism [7], group 2 included patients with both findings.

Statistical data analysis was done by odds ratio as well as X^2 testing using Yates' correction for small numbers when mandatory.

Results

196 (98%) patients completed the study. The 4 missing cases had magnetic resonance tomography or no investigation for clinical reasons.

ECHO results are shown in table 2. 189 patients were submitted to both a transesophageal and a transthoracic approach (7 to only one of the approaches). A total of 27 thrombi were seen in 26 patients. Five of these thrombi were in the atrium and could only be detected by transesophageal ECHO. Furthermore, a large number of other presumed sources of embolism emerged, the most frequent being mitral-valve prolapse (n = 58) and hypokinetic wall segments (n = 45). Many cases showed more than one source of embolism.

ECG showed 23 cases with atrial fibrillation (AF), including 2 with atrial flutter and another 2 with intermittent AF. Only 1 individual with AF also had an atrial thrombus.

Doppler sonography and B-scan revealed 28 carotid-artery stenoses (> 50%) ipsilateral to the classifying event and another 21 contralateral carotid-artery stenoses, most of them in combination with one of the 28 ipsilateral stenoses. Significant vertebral-artery stenoses could not be detected.

Table 2. Cardiac sources of embolism in transthoracic and transesophageal echocardiography in 196 ischemic stroke patients[1]

Source of embolism	n	%
Thrombus – total[2]	27	13.8
Left atrium[3]	5	2.6
Left ventricle	22	11.2
Mitral valve prolapse	58	29.6
Atrial septum aneurysm	29	14.8
Pseudoaneurysm[3]	3	1.5
Patent foramen ovale[3]	16	8.2
Septum defect[3]	7	3.6
Hypokinetic wall segment	45	23.0
Endocarditis	1	0.5
Hypertrophic, obstructive cardiomyopathy	2	1.0

[1] 189 patients with both the transthoracic and transesophageal approach; 7 patients with one approach only.
[2] One patient with both atrial and ventricular thrombus.
[3] Exclusively found by transesophageal echocardiography.

Table 3. CCT in 196 ischemic stroke patients

Type	Ischemic lesions	
	n	%
Pial-artery infarcts (PAI)	71	36.2
Lacunes	51	26.0
Low-flow infarcts (LF)	16	8.2
Unclassified	17	8.7
Normal	68	34.7
Subgroup: combined infarct patterns – total	25	12.8
Lacunes + PAI	10	5.1
LF + PAI	5	2.6
PAI + unclassified	4	2.0
LF + lacunes	3	1.5
LF + unclassified	1	0.5
PAI + LF + lacune	1	0.5
PAI + lacune + unclassified	1	0.5

Note that patients could have more than one lesion pattern – as sown in the subgroup of combined patterns – which causes the numbers to exceed the total of 196 investigations.

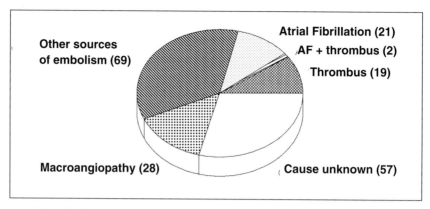

Fig. 1. Etiological stroke factors in 196 ischemic stroke patients.

CCT results are given in table 3. The majority of lesions seen were either of the pial-artery (71 cases) or the lacunar (51 cases) type. A total of 25 patients showed a combination of two or more infarct patterns with lacunes and pial-artery infarcts as the most frequently coexisting lesions. Low-flow infarcts were less frequent (16 cases). In 17 cases, lesions were rated as 'unclassified', and another 68 patients had normal CCT scans.

According to the sonographic (ECHO, Doppler sonography) and ECG findings, the patients were assigned to the following three groups (fig. 1): Group 1 (cardiac sources of embolism, no signs of macroangiopathy) contained more than half (n = 111) of all patients: AF in 21 cases; thrombi in 19 (4 in the left atrium, and 16 in the left ventricle, including 1 patient with thrombi in both compartments). Two additional cases presented with both AF and a cardiac thrombus (1 atrial, 1 ventricular). 69 patients had other sources of embolism, either single or combined. Group 2 (macroangiopathy) comprised 28 patients with carotid-artery stenoses (> 50%, ipsilateral to the classifying event). 21 of these cases showed an additional cardiac source of embolism (5 ventricular thrombi, 2 AF, 14 other sources). The remaining 57 patients (group 3) disclosed no cardiac sources of embolism or carotid stenoses and could be subdivided into 35 cases with and 22 without hypertension.

The observed frequencies of CCT patterns in groups 1–3 are given in table 4. Statistical data analysis was first done for the total number of

Table 4. CCT patterns and possible stroke mechanisms in 196 patients

| | CCT pattern | | | | | |
	PAI	LAC	LF	COMB	UC	normal
All lesions	71	51	16	25	17	68
Subgroups:						
Fresh lesions	57	23	8		5	
Multiple lesions	8	19	2		0	
Group 1: Cardiac sources of embolism – total (n = 111)						
All lesions	42	29	7	16[1]	9	42
Fresh lesions	31	10	2		2	
Multiple lesions	7	7	0			
Group 1a: Thrombus (n = 21)[2]						
All	9	5	2	6*	3	8
Fresh	8	1	0		0	
Multiple	1	1	0			
Group 1b: AF (n = 23)[2]						
All	12	5	1	3	1	7
Fresh	9	2	1		0	
Multiple	3**	1	0			
Group 1c: Other sources (n = 69)[3]						
All	22	20	4	81	5	28
Fresh	15	7	1		2	
Multiple	3	5	0			
Group 2: Macroangiopathy (n = 28)						
All	12	7	5	5	3	6
Fresh	11	3	4***		2	
Multiple	0	4	2			
Group 3 (n = 57): No cardiac source, no macroangiopathy						
All	17	15	4	4	5	20
Fresh	15	10	2		1	
Multiple	1	8	0			

PAI = Pial-artery infarct; LAC = lacune; LF = low-flow infarct; COMB = combined lesion patterns; UC = unclassified.
[1] Two patients with three types of infarcts.
[2] The AF and thrombus groups overlap in 2 patients.
[3] Other sources of embolism: mitral valve prolapse, hypokinetic myocardial wall, septum aneurysm, patent foramen ovale, atrial septum defect, endocarditis.
*   Odds ratio 3.28 (1.14–9.46), $p < 0.05$ X^2.
**   Odds ratio 5.04 (1.12–22.65).
***   Odds ratio 6.83 (1.60–29.10), $p < 0.05$ X^2.

Table 5. Frequency of lacunes in hypertensive versus non-hypertensive cases with no cardiac source of embolism or macroangiopathy

	Lacunes	Other lesions[1]
Hypertensive patients (n = 35)	10	25
Non-hypertensive patients (n = 22)	5	17

Statistics (X^2 cross-tabulation): no significant difference.
[1] Including normal CCT scans.

each ischemic lesion pattern in the three groups. In support of the null hypothesis, there was no significant difference between the observed and the expected frequencies of pial-artery, lacunar and low-flow infarcts. It was only in small subgroups that significant differences emerged: patients with multiple pial-artery infarcts more often disclosed AF ($p < 0.05$); fresh low-flow infarcts coincided with carotid-artery stenoses ($p < 0.05$), and combined CCT patterns were more often accompanied by cardiac thrombi ($p < 0.05$). Finally, even in the absence of cardiac sources of embolism and/or macroangiopathy, CCT did not reveal significantly more lacunes in hypertensive than in non-hypertensive patients (table 5).

As a post hoc defined subgroup, CCT patterns of 7 patients with extracranial carotid-artery stenoses and no additional cardiac source of embolism were analyzed. Three of these cases showed low-flow, 2 pial-artery infarcts, 1 a lacune, and 1 a normal CCT.

Conclusions

In general, the association of CCT patterns with possible stroke mechanisms was weak. CCT in patients with cardiac sources of embolism show a variety of morphological patterns including lacunes. The predictive value of CCT patterns for the finding of cardiac sources of embolism or extracranial macroangiopathy is low and restricted to the subgroup of low-flow infarcts. Classification systems of stroke etiology should allow different CCT patterns in each etiological category. Regardless of the CCT pattern a complete cardiovascular sonographic investigation is necessary in every case of cerebral ischemia.

Zusammenfassung

Computertomographische Muster zerebraler Ischämien bei Patienten mit kardialen Emboliequellen, extrakranieller Makroangiopathie oder fehlendem Hinweis auf eine extrakranielle Schlaganfallursache

In einer prospektiven Studie sollte die Frage einer Assoziation zwischen Hirninfarkt-mechanismen (kardiogene Embolie, extrakranielle Makroangiopathie, hypertensive Mikroangiopathie) und CCT-morphologischen Befunden untersucht werden.

200 konsekutive Patienten mit fokalen zerebralen Ischämien wurden mit Echokardiographie (transthorakal und transösophageal), Doppler-Sonographie, EKG und CCT untersucht. Die Auswertung der CCT-Bilder erfolgte blind, d. h. dem Untersucher waren die klinischen und anderen apparativen Ergebnisse unbekannt.

Außer einer Assoziation zwischen Grenzzoneninfarkten und Karotisstenosen ließen sich keine klaren Korrelationen von Hirninfarktmechanismen und CCT-Mustern finden. Lakunare Infarktmuster im CCT zeigten sich mit fast gleicher Häufigkeit bei Patienten mit kardialen Emboliequellen, extrakranieller Makroangiopathie oder fehlendem Hinweis auf extrakranielle Infarktursachen. Hypertonie und lakunare Infarktmuster waren ebenfalls nicht miteinander assoziiert.

Der prädiktive Wert von CCT-Mustern für positive Befunde bei der Suche nach spezifischen extrakraniellen Hirninfarktursachen ist gering. Eine embolische Genese von lakunaren Läsionen im CCT kann nicht ausgeschlossen werden.

References

1   Ringelstein EB, Koschorke S, Holling A, Thron A, Lambertz H, Minale C: Computed tomographic patterns of proven embolic brain infarctions. Ann Neurol 1989;26:759–765.
2   Mohr JP, Barnett HJM: Classification of ischemic strokes; in Barnett HJM, Mohr JP, Stein BM, Yatsu FM (eds): Stroke, Pathophysiology, Diagnosis, and Management. New York, Churchill Livingstone, 1986, pp 281–291.
3   Ringelstein EB, Weiller C: Hirninfarktmuster im Computertomogramm: Pathophysiologische Konzepte, Validierung und klinische Relevanz. Nervenarzt 1990;61:462–471.
4   Horowitz DR, Tuhrim S, Weinberger JM, Rudolph SH: Mechanisms in lacunar infarction. Stroke 1992;23:325–327.
5   Millikan C, Futrell N: The fallacy of the lacune hypothesis. Stroke 1990;21:1251–1257.
6   Foulkes MA, Wolf PA, Price TR, Mohr JP, Hier DB: The Stroke Data Bank: Design, methods, and baseline characteristics. Unpublished extended version of: Foulkes MA, Wolf PA, Price TR, Mohr JP, Hier DB: The Stroke Data Bank: Design, methods, and baseline characteristics. Stroke 1988;19:547–554. 1987; manuscript BFSB 87101.
7   Weinberger J, Rothlauf E, Materese E, Halperin J: Noninvasive evaluation of the extracranial carotid arteries in patients with cerebrovascular events and atrial fibrillation. Arch Intern Med 1988;148:1785.
8   Russo LS: Letter to the editor. Stroke 1992;23:1032.

9   Hart RG, Sherman DG, Miller VT: Diagnosis and management of ischemic stroke. II. Selected controversies. Curr Probl Cardiol 1983;8:71–77.
10 Sandercock PAG, Warlow CP, Jones LN, Starkey IR: Predisposing factors for cerebral infarction: The Oxfordshire community stroke project. Br Med J 1989;298:75–80.
11 Cerebral Embolism Task Force: Cardiogenic brain embolism. Arch Neurol 1986;43:71–84.
12 Wolf PA, Abbott RD, Kannel WB: Atrial fibrillation as an independent risk factor for stroke: The Framingham Study. Stroke 1991;22:983–988.
13 Van Merwijk G, Lodder J, Bamford J, Kester ADM: How often is non-valvular atrial fibrillation the cause of brain infarction? J Neurol 1990;237:205–207.

Dr. H. Mast
Abteilung Neurologie
Universitätsklinikum Steglitz
der Freien Universität Berlin
Hindenburgdamm 30
D-12200 Berlin (FRG)

Dorndorf W, Marx P (eds): Stroke Prevention.
Basel, Karger, 1994, pp 37–44

Predictive Value of Major Risk Factors and the Impact of Their Control

H. C. Diener

Department of Neurology, University of Essen, FRG

The term risk factor is used for the purpose of this article as physiological characteristics and behaviors that predict future occurrence of stroke. The following risk factors will be covered: hypertension, lipids, smoking, alcohol, diabetes mellitus and estrogen replacement. The three main classes of stroke – ischemic stroke, intracranial hemorrhage and subarachnoidal hemorrhage – are not considered separately in most studies. This may explain the sometimes conflicting results of epidemiological or preventive studies.

Hypertension

Hypertension is the most important risk factor for stroke. The relative risk of stroke in patients with hypertension varies between 2.5 and 6.3 [3, 21]. The risk of stroke increases with both the systolic and diastolic blood pressure [23]. MacMahon et al. [11] performed a meta-analysis from 9 prospective trials involving 420,000 people: 843 strokes occurred during the 10-year follow-up period. The risk of stroke was linearly related to diastolic blood pressure within a range of 75–105 mm Hg. The absolute risk was larger for coronary heart disease than for stroke.

Collins et al. [5] examined in a second overview 14 randomized trials of antihypertensive drugs in 37,000 individuals. The mean treatment duration was 5 years. The reduction in risk of stroke was 42% (fig. 1) but only 14% for coronary heart disease. Most of the earlier studies involved middle-aged subjects. Two recent trials investigated whether the treatment of hypertension is able to prevent stroke in the elderly [6, 16] (see table 1).

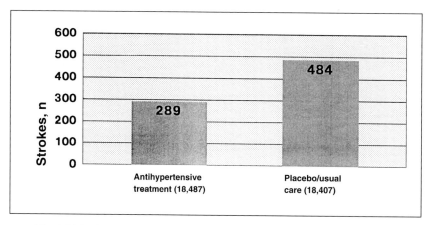

Fig. 1. Risk of stroke (number of strokes) in patients on antihypertensive treatment and on placebo. The relative risk reduction is 42% [data from 5].

Table 1. Reduction in the risk of stroke by antihypertensive treatment in the elderly (STOP and SHEP trials)

	Study			
	STOP		SHEP	
Participants	1,627		4,736	
Sex, % females	63		57	
Mean age, years	75.6		72	
Inclusion criteria				
Age, years	> 70		> 60	
RR systolic, mm Hg	> 180		> 160	
RR diastolic, mm Hg	≥ 90		< 90	
Follow-up, months	65		48–60	
Therapy I	β-blockers		diuretics	
	diuretics		atenolol	
Therapy II	placebo		placebo	
Endpoints	stroke, myocardial		stroke, myocardial	
	infarction (MI),		infarction, mortality,	
	vascular death		quality of living	
	Results, n			
	therapy	placebo	therapy	placebo
Stroke	29	35*	103	159*
MI	25	28	62	82*
Death	36	63*	213	242*

* Significant differences.

In terms of costs, risks and benefit, one has to consider how many patients with hypertension have to be treated to prevent one stroke. These numbers are 170 for the MRC trial [13], 33 for SHEP and 14 for STOP. The preventive effect of antihypertensive treatment was however only shown for diuretics and β-blockers (metoprolol, propranolol and atenolol). Calcium antagonists and ACE inhibitors were not investigated in this respect.

Lipids

The relation between serum cholesterol and stroke is not clear. Cholesterol is possibly not an independent risk factor for stroke [15, 21]. The American multiple risk factor intervention trial [10] measured serum cholesterol and stroke mortality in 350,977 men. The risk of stroke was increased above a cholesterol level of 240 mg/dl (fig. 2). A meta-analysis by Muldoon et al. [14] included 24,847 male participants with a mean age of 47.5 years. During the 119,000 person-years, 1,147 deaths occurred. The analysis revealed a decrease in mortality from heart disease with lowering cholesterol concentrations, but total mortality was not affected by treatment.

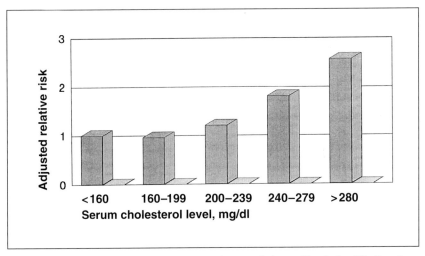

Fig. 2. Adjusted relative risk of stroke and serum cholesterol levels (mg/dl). Data from 350,977 men [data from 10].

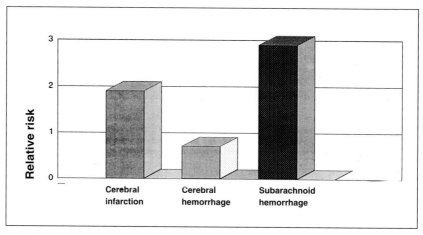

Fig. 3. Cigarette smoking and stroke [data from 17].

Smoking

Smoking is a risk factor for stroke. A review of the literature by Dal Bianco et al. [7] and a meta-analysis of 32 prospective risk factor studies by Shinton and Beevers [17] found a relative risk of stroke with smoking between 1.5 and 2 (fig. 3). The risk is higher for cerebral infarction and subarachnoid hemorrhage compared to cerebral hemorrhage, higher for females compared to men, and increases with the number of cigarettes per day. The influence of cessation of smoking was investigated in several observational studies. The risk reduction for myocardial infarction after stopping smoking is 50–70% [12]; the risk reduction for stroke is not known.

Alcohol

Although heavy alcohol use has been shown to increase the risk of stroke [9], there is evidence from epidemiologic studies to suggest that moderate consumption of alcohol reduces the risk of ischemic stroke [8, 20]. There is, however, a linear relationship between alcohol intake and the risk of cerebral and subarachnoid hemorrhage [4, 8].

Noninsulin-Dependent Diabetes mellitus

In population-based studies, the age-adjusted morbidity and mortality rates for stroke are two times higher among diabetics [1, 2, 22]. The risk profile is confounded by additional risk factors like obesity and lack of physical activity. The influence of maintaining strict glycemic control either by diet or drug treatment on stroke among patients with diabetes mellitus remains uncertain.

Postmenopausal Estrogen Replacement Therapy

The use of oral contraceptives in premenopausal women is associated with an increased risk of stroke [18]. Endogenous estrogens have a major role in the low risk of heart disease and stroke observed in premenopausal women, because after menopause the risk begins to increase. A recent study by Stampfer et al. [19] investigated the influence of postmenopausal estrogen replacement in a 10-year follow-up study in 48,470 women. During the observation period, 224 strokes and 405 major coronary events occurred. The relative risk of a major coronary disease was 0.56 and the relative risk for stroke was 0.97 in women taking estrogen compared to women without estrogen replacement.

Conclusions

A number of risk factors is clearly related with the risk of stroke (table 2). Intervention trials to show the benefit of the treatment of a par-

Table 2. Summary of risk factors and stroke

	Relative risk	Intervention trials
Hypertension	+++	++
Smoking	++	–
Alcohol	++	–
Cholesterol	?	–
Diabetes	?	–
Obesity	?	–

ticular risk factor are only available for the treatment of hypertension. A number of interventions however may at least reduce the risk of a major cardial event.

Zusammenfassung

Prädiktiver Wert der wichtigsten Risikofaktoren und der Einfluß ihrer Kontrolle

Der Terminus Risikofaktor wird in dieser Arbeit als Merkmal definiert, das die Wahrscheinlichkeit eines in der Zukunft eintretenden Schlaganfalles vorhersagt. Im einzelnen soll auf folgende Risikofaktoren eingegangen werden: Hypertonie, Hyperlipidämie, Rauchen, Alkohol, nicht insulinabhängiger Diabetes mellitus und postmenopausale Östrogensubstitution.

Hypertonie: Dies ist der wichtigste Risikofaktor für Schlaganfälle. Das relative Risiko steigt mit Hypertonie um einen Faktor von 2,5 bis 6,3, und zwar bei Erhöhung sowohl des systolischen als auch des diastolischen Blutdrucks. In einer Metaanalyse [Lancet 1990;335:765–774] von neun prospektiven Untersuchungen an 420 000 Probanden war das Schlaganfallrisiko linear mit einem diastolischen Blutdruck von zwischen 75 und 105 mm Hg korreliert. Das absolute Risiko war für Herzinfarkte größer als für Schlaganfälle. Eine andere Studie [Lancet 1990;335:827–838] unterzog 14 randomisierte Untersuchungen (37 000 Patienten) über die protektive Wirksamkeit einer antihypertensiven Therapie einer Metaanalyse. Bei einer durchschnittlichen Behandlungsdauer von 5 Jahren konnten 42% der Schlaganfälle, aber nur 14% der Herzinfarkte verhindert werden. Ähnliche Ergebnisse fanden sich auch bei zwei jüngeren Untersuchungen an alten Menschen: dem STOP Trial [Lancet 1991;338:1281–1285] und der Arbeit der SHEP Cooperative Research Group [JAMA 1991;265:3255–3264]. Beim MRC Trial [Br Med J 1985;291:97–104] mußten 170, bei SHEP 33 und beim STOP Trial 14 Patienten behandelt werden, um einen Schlaganfall zu verhindern.

Hyperlipidämie: Cholesterin ist möglicherweise kein unabhängiger Risikofaktor für ischämische Insulte. Der American Multiple Risk Factor Intervention Trial [N Engl J Med 1989;320:904–910] zeigte allerdings bei 350 977 Männern eine Schlaganfallrisikoerhöhung bei Werten von über 240 mg/dl. Eine Metaanalyse [Br Med J 1990;301:309–314] ergab bei 24 847 männlichen Teilnehmern (119 000 Patientenjahre) eine Verminderung der Sterblichkeit an kardialen Erkrankungen durch eine Senkung des Cholesterinwertes. Die Gesamtmortalität war jedoch nicht beeinflußt.

Rauchen: Eine Literaturübersicht [Akt Neurol 1988;15:15–21] und eine Metaanalyse von 32 prospektiven Untersuchungen [Br Med J 1989;298:789–794) ergaben ein relatives Risiko von 1,5 bis 2. Das Risiko ist für ischämische Insulte und Subarachnoidalblutungen höher als für Hirnblutungen. Die Risikoreduktion durch Abstinenz beläuft sich für Myokardinfarkte auf 50–70%, für ischämische Insulte ist sie nicht bekannt.

Alkohol: Starker Alkoholkonsum erhöht das Risiko für Schlaganfälle [Acta Med Scand 1987 (Suppl 717):93–106]. Epidemiologische Studien legen allerdings die Annahme nahe, daß leichter Alkoholkonsum das Risiko ischämischer Insulte verringert [Am J Med

1991;90:489–497; N Engl J Med 1988:319;267–273]. Unabhängig davon besteht jedoch eine lineare Beziehung zwischen Alkoholkonsum und intrazerebralen und subarachnoidalen Blutungen [Stroke 1989;20:1611–1626].

Nicht insulinabhängiger Diabetes mellitus: Bevölkerungsstudien [JAMA 1987;257: 949–952; Am J Epidemiol 1988;128:116–123; Stroke 1991;22:312–318] zeigen, daß die alterskorrigierten Erkrankungs- und Sterblichkeitsraten für Schlaganfälle bei Diabetikern doppelt so hoch sind wie bei Nichtdiabetikern. Die Aussage ist jedoch durch begleitende Parameter, wie Übergewicht und Mangel an physischer Tätigkeit, eingeschränkt. Der Einfluß der Diabeteseinstellung auf die Schlaganfallrate ist nicht bekannt.

Postmenopausale Östrogensubstitution: Oral verabreichte Kontrazeptiva erhöhen das Schlaganfallrisiko [N Engl J Med 1981;305:612–618]. Die endogene Östrogenproduktion hat hingegen offenbar einen protektiven Effekt in Hinblick auf koronare Erkrankungen und Schlaganfälle. Eine Untersuchung [N Engl J Med 1991;325:756–762] zeigte, daß postmenopausale Östrogensubstitution bei 48 470 Frauen über einen Beobachtungszeitraum von 10 Jahren mit einem relativen Risiko für schwere kardiale Erkrankungen von 0,56 und auf einem für Schlaganfälle von 0,97 verbunden war.

Insgesamt haben die bisherigen Untersuchungen einige Risikofaktoren für Schlaganfälle klar identifizieren können. Positive Resultate von Interventionsstudien liegen in bezug auf Schlaganfälle bisher nur für die Hypertonie vor.

References

1   Abbott RD, Donahue RP, MacMahon SW, Reed DM, Yano K: Diabetes and the risk of stroke. The Honolulu Heart Program. J Am Med Assoc 1987;257:949–952.

2   Barrett-Connor E, Khaw K: Diabetes mellitus: An independent risk factor for stroke. Am J Epidemiol 1988;128:116–123.

3   Bonita R, Beaglehole R: Does treatment of hypertension explain the decline in mortality from stroke? Br Med J 1986; 292:191–192.

4   Camargo CA: Moderate alcohol consumption and stroke. The epidemiologic evidence. Stroke 1989;20:1611–1626.

5   Collins R, Peto R, MacMahon S, Hebert P, Fiebach NH, Eberlein KA, Godwin J, Qizilbash N, Taylor JO, Hennekens CH: Blood pressure, stroke and coronary heart disease. 2. Short-term reductions in blood pressure: overview of randomized drug trials in their epidemiological context. Lancet 1990;335:827–838.

6   Dahlöf B, Lindholm LH, Hansson L, Schersten B, Ekbom T, Wester P-O: Morbidity and mortality in the Swedish trial in old patients with hypertension (STOP hypertension). Lancet 1991;338:1281–1285.

7   Dal Bianco P, Zeiler K, Auff E, Baumgartner C, Holzner F, Deecke L: Zigarettenkonsum und Schlaganfall. Akt Neurol 1988;15:15–21.

8   Gill JS, Shipley MJ, Tsementzis SA, Hornby RS, Gill SK, Hitchcock ER, Beevers DG: Alcohol consumption – A risk factor for hemorrhagic and non-hemorrhagic stroke. Am J Med 1991;90:489–497.

9   Hillbom ME: What supports the role of alcohol as a risk factor for stroke? Acta Med Scand 1987(Suppl 717):93–106.

10 Iso H, Jacobs DR, Wentworth D, Neaton JD, Cohen JD: Serum cholesterol levels and six-year mortality from stroke in 350,977 men screened for the multiple risk factor intervention trial. N Engl J Med 1989;320:904–910.

11 MacMahon S, Peto R, Cutler J, Collins R, Sorlie P, Neaton J, Abbott R, Godwin J, Dyer A, Stamler J: Blood pressure, stroke and coronary heart disease. 1. Prolonged differences in blood pressure: prospective observational studies corrected for the regression dilution bias. Lancet 1990;335:765–774.

12 Manson JE, Tosteson H, Ridker PM, Satterfield S, Hebert P, O'Connor GT, Buring JE, Hennekens CH: The primary prevention of myocardial infarction. N Engl J Med 1992;326:1406–1416.

13 Medical Research Council Working Party: MRC trial of treatment of mild hypertension: Principal results. Br Med J 1985;291:97–104.

14 Muldoon MF, Manuck SB, Matthews KA: Lowering cholesterol concentrations and mortality: A quantitative review of primary prevention trials. Br Med J 1990;301:309–314.

15 Shaper AG, Phillips AN, Pocock SJ, Walker M, Macfarlane PW: Risk factors for stroke in middle-aged British men. Br Med J 1991;302:1111–1115.

16 SHEP Cooperative Research Group: Prevention of stroke by antihypertensive drug treatment in older persons with isolated systolic hypertension. J Am Med Assoc 1991; 265:3255–3264.

17 Shinton R, Beevers G: Meta-analysis of relation between cigarette smoking and stroke. Br Med J 1989;298:789–794.

18 Stadel BV: Oral contraceptives and cardiovascular disease. N Engl J Med 1981;305:612–618.

19 Stampfer MJ, Colditz GA, Willett WC, Manson JE, Rosner B, Speizer FE, Hennekens CH: Postmenopausal estrogen therapy and cardiovascular disease. Ten-year follow-up from the Nurses' Health Study. N Engl J Med 1991;325:756–762.

20 Stampfer MJ, Colditz GA, Willett WC, Speizer FE, Hennekens CH: A prospective study of moderate alcohol consumption and the risk of coronary disease and stroke in women. N Engl J Med 1988;319:267–273.

21 Welin L, Svaerdsudd K, Wilhelmsen L, Larsson B: Analysis of risk factors for stroke in a cohort of men born in 1913. N Engl J Med 1987;317:521–526.

22 Wolf PA, D'Agostino B, Belanger AJ, Kannel WB: Probability of stroke: A risk profile from the Framingham study. Stroke 1991;22:312–318.

23 Wolf PA, Kannel WB, McGee DL: Prevention of ischemic stroke: risk factors. Barnett HJM, Stein BM, Mohr JP, Yatsu FM (eds.): In: Stroke. pp 967–988. Churchill Livingstone, New York 1986.

Prof. Dr. H. C. Diener
Department of Neurology
University of Essen
Hufelandstraße 55
D-45122 Essen (FRG)

Dorndorf W, Marx P (eds): Stroke Prevention.
Basel, Karger, 1994, pp 45–52

Transient Ischemic Attacks in Baboons due to Platelet Microemboli[1]

*Christof M. Kessler[a], Andrew B. Kelly[b], William D. Suggs[c],
Steven R. Hanson[b], Laurence A. Harker[b]*

[a] Department of Neurology, Medizinische Universität zu Lübeck, FRG
[b] Division of Hematology and Oncology, and
[c] Department of Surgery, Emory University School of Medicine, Atlanta, Ga., USA

Platelet emboli from atherosclerotic lesions in extracranial arteries frequently cause cerebral ischemia [1–3]. Measurements of blood markers of thrombosis during the acute phase of stroke enables to recognize patients with an ongoing thrombotic process. Since acute stroke therapy must aim at a rapid dissolution of the embolized thrombi, adequate animal models are required to test future clinical applications of different drug regimens. As the vascular anatomy, coagulation system, fibrinolytic system, and pharmacokinetics of nonhuman primates are most similar to man [4–6], they are useful as a model for cerebrovascular disease in humans. We developed a model of stroke in baboons using endogenously produced platelet emboli that produces transient neurological deficits and enables to study the preciseness of thrombosis marker estimation as well as the quantification of embolized amount of platelet emboli.

Material and Methods

Four juvenile male baboons *(Papio cynocephalus)* weighing 12–18 kg were used. They were observed for at least 6 weeks to ensure that they were free of any diseases. All experiments were performed in compliance with the 'Principles of Laboratory Animal Care' and

[1] Supported in part by grants HL 31950, HL 41619, HL 31469 and RR 00165 from the National Institutes of Health. C.M.K. was a visiting scientist supported by a grant of the Deutsche Forschungsgemeinschaft.

the 'Guide for Care and Use of Laboratory Animals' (NIH Production No. 80–23, revised 1985).

The initial platelet counts averaged at 331,000 ± 57,900 platelets/µl; the mean white cell count was 5,330 ± 1580 cells/µl and the mean hematocrit was 33.5 ± 2.1%. While general anesthesia was induced with ketamine HCl (20 mg/kg) and halothane (1–2%) in oxygen via an endotracheal tube, one carotid artery was isolated and a 75-cm long nonthrombogenic arterio-arterial (A–A) shunt of 3 mm i. d. (Dow Corning Corp., Midland, Mich., USA) silicone rubber tubing was inserted in the common carotid artery. Flow was re-established with a roller pump (Masterflex; Cole Parmer, Chicago, Ill., USA) at a flow rate of 80 ml/min. Endogenous platelet microemboli were generated by a 40-cm thrombogenic Dacron graft device of 4 mm i. d. (US Catheter Inc., Billerica, Mass., USA) inserted into the arterial-arterial shunt for 1 h, while the A-A shunt was retained in place for another hour. Before inserting the A-A shunt, autologous baboon platelets were labeled with ^{111}In oxide according to a previously described protocol [7], and 1.5 mCi were injected intravenously. Scintigraphic images of the brain were recorded in a flexed posterior-anterior position with a General Electric 400 T MaxiCamera (General Electric Co., Milwaukee, Wisc., USA) interfaced with a Medical Data System and A^2 image processing computer (Medtronic, Ann Arbor, Mich., USA) using a medium-energy collimator. Images of the brain were recorded in 5-min sequences, additionally the ^{111}In activity of 4-ml samples whole blood (blood standard) and the vascular graft devices removed from circulation was recorded.

The total platelet count (labeled plus unlabeled) of each hemisphere was calculated as previously described [8] with the ^{111}In activity of both hemispheric regions of interest (ROI), the ^{111}In activity of the standards, and the platelet counts. Passing carotid platelet microemboli were registered by continuous transcranial Doppler monitoring (Transspect TCD; Medasonics, Fermont, Calif., USA) in the affected carotid artery via the transorbital window. The Doppler beam was focused on 4.5 cm depth with a 2-MHz probe.

After surgically closing the carotid artery shunt sites, 2 animals were recovered and their neurological function was assessed using a nonhuman primate disability score [9] at 60 min and 12 and 24 h. The remaining animals underwent a pressure perfusion fixation [10], and their brain cuts were stained with hematoxylin and eosin for light microscopical examination. Before and 60 and 120 min after inserting the graft, platelet and white cell counts as well as fibrinogen levels, activated partial thromboplastin time (APTT), fibrinopeptide A (FP-A), β-thromboglobulin (β-TG), and platelet factor 4 (PF-4) were measured. Fibrinogen was estimated as total thrombin clotable protein [10], APTT using Thrombosil I (Ortho Diagnostic Systems, Raritan, N. J., USA). In 3 animals, the levels of β-TG, PF-4, and FP-A were estimated as thrombosis markers. β-TG was measured by a commercially available radioimmunoassay (Amersham, Arlington Heights, Ill., USA) as well as PF-4 (Abbott Laboratories, Chicago, Ill., USA). The FP-A levels were measured as described elsewere [11].

Results

Immediately after establishing the blood flow through the thrombogenic Dacron vascular graft extension into the A-A shunt, the transorbital transcranial Doppler registered continuously microemboli passing through

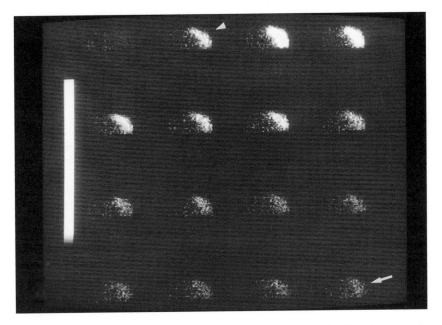

Fig. 1. Sixteen gamma camera images in 10-min sequences. After inserting the graft, platelets accumulate in the left hemisphere (arrowhead) and spontaneously clear within 160 min (arrow).

the carotid artery. Coincidently, the scintigraphic images documented a rapid accumulation of ^{111}In platelets in the ipsilateral cerebral hemisphere (fig. 1). The mean hemispheric baseline platelet value was $0.36 \pm 0.11 \times 10^9$ platelets, but the maximum value within 20 min counted $3.2 \pm 11 \times 10^9$ platelets ($p < 0.001$).

Thereafter the amount of platelet microemboli falls in the affected carotid territory to $1.30 \pm 0.4 \times 10^9$ platelets 40 min later, despite the fact that the thrombogenic vascular graft was still inserted. After removing the grafts, ^{111}In platelets continued to clear from the cerebral circulation and reached the basal value at $0.48 \pm 0.13 \times 10^9$ 60 min later. No changes of ^{111}In platelet activities were observed in the nonembolized contralateral hemisphere.

There was no change in hematocrit, white cell counts and fibrinogen levels during the experiment. Within the first hour the mean peripheral platelet count dropped at 25.3% from $331,000 \pm 57,900$ to $247,00 \pm 45,600$ due to the platelet consumption in the graft. Table 1

Table 1. Blood markers of thrombosis

	Pregraft	Postgraft	
		60 min	120 min
β-TG, ng/ml	6.9 ± 1.7	127.0 ± 51.6	33.3 ± 12.1
PF-4, ng/ml	7.3 ± 0.6	54.0 ± 3.9	10.8 ± 4.0
FP-A, nmol/ml	3.4 ± 1.6	32.1 ± 2.8	2.3 ± 1.2
APTT, s	53.9 ± 21.6	86.2 ± 12.4	70.5 ± 2.3

shows the values of β-TG, PF-4, FP-A and APTT: they all significantly increased during the first hour after the insertion of the graft. After a 2-hour period, PF-4, FP-A and β-TG dropped to nearly initial values, but APTT decreased only slightly.

After recovering from anesthesia, the animals exhibited a mild contralateral hemiparesis including a facial paresis (clinical score of 54 and 35 compared with basal score of 100). Twelve hours later the animals were normal in motor and cranial nerve function as well as in behavior (both a clinical score of 100). The neuropathological examination of pressure-perfused brains exhibited normal vessels without evidence for thrombotic occlusion of the intracerebral arteries, except for a single thrombus found in a superficial meningeal vessel.

Discussion

We demonstrated that platelet emboli temporarily retained in the affected carotid territories produce transient neurological symptoms that resolve many hours after the platelet emboli clear from the hemispheric circulation. During the embolization, both the markers of platelet activation as well as of coagulation increased substantially, but normalized rapidly afterwards. Since platelet emboli arising from carotid atherosclerotic lesions are a common cause of transient ischemic attacks (TIA) and stroke [1, 2] our quantitative model of cerebral microembolization is useful to evaluate novel acute stroke therapies.

Several stroke models have been described in nonhuman primates [9–11]. They have employed either acute mechanical occlusion of the middle cerebral artery or embolization with microspheres. Those approaches obviously do not reflect the interactions between vessel wall and platelet emboli which are important pathophysiological variables. In our model, ^{111}In labeling of platelets enables us to quantify and localize embolized platelet aggregates during the perfusion time. In addition, transcranial Doppler proved pathing formed emboli during the incorporation time of the segments of vascular graft, whereas the absence of detectable microemboli before graft insertion proved that the A-A carotid shunt did not contribute as a source of microembolization.

The generation of platelet emboli by vascular graft segments incorporated into A-A shunts in baboons has been previously demonstrated [12, 13]. After inserting the graft, a significant drop of circulating platelet count was observed, which proves the platelet consumption by the graft segment. The plasma levels of all measured thrombosis markers increased significantly, thus revealing the simultaneous involvement of the coagulation system. The exposure of the graft to flowing blood results in a significant fall of circulating platelet count by one fourth due to platelet consumption by the graft. Gamma camera images illustrated a rapid accumulation of embolized platelets but also a subsequent disappearance of hemispheric embolized platelets. However, in a previous study on a peripheral artery embolic model in baboons, Schneider et al. [12] demonstrated retention of ^{111}In platelet emboli in the vascular circulation of the leg for many hours; thus, only 25% of platelet emboli in the leg are cleared during a 4-hour period. This difference in retention of platelet emboli by different vascular beds shows different protecting mechanisms of the cerebral circulation, e. g. embolus-initiated vasodilatation or a more rapid embolus disruption by better availability of prostacyclin or nitric oxide [14, 15] may contribute in these processes. Clearance of microemboli from the cerebral circulation is confirmed by neuropathology, demonstrating an absence of embolized material. The full recovery of neurological function in awake animals after initial transient neurological symptoms contralaterally to the embolized cerebral hemisphere shows that embolized platelet microparticles produce transient cerebral dysfunction. In a previous report, we could also demonstrate abolishing and subsequent recovery of somatosensory evoked potential ipsilateral to the embolic carotid territory.

In summary, our quantitative model of hemispheric embolization with endogenously generated platelet aggregates produces experimental transient neurological symptoms and may be useful for the examination of pathophysiology and therapeutic interventions in embolic stroke.

Zusammenfassung

Flüchtige ischämische Attacken durch Mikroemboli bei Pavianen

Plättchenembolien von arteriosklerotischen Gefäßveränderungen verursachen oft zerebrale Ischämien [Stroke, Philadelphia, Lea & Febiger, 1987, pp 48–52; Q J Med 1964;33:155–195; Arch Neurol 1986;43:71–84]. Gleichzeitig lassen sich während akuten Schlaganfallphasen Veränderungen der Koagulationsparameter im Blut nachweisen.

Wir stellen ein Tiermodell bei Pavianen zur Untersuchung der Pathophysiologie und der Behandlung von Plättchenembolien vor, deren Gefäßanatomie, Gerinnungs- und Fibrinolysesystem sowie Pharmakokinetik den Verhältnissen beim Menschen ähnlich sind. Vier junge Paviane mit einem Gewicht von 12 bis 18 kg wurden benutzt. Unter Ketamin- und Halothannarkose wurde eine Karotisarterie isoliert und ein 75 cm langer, nicht thrombogener arterio-arterieller Shunt aus Silikon mit einem inneren Durchmesser von 3 mm eingepflanzt. Der Blutfluß wurde über eine Rollerpumpe wiederhergestellt. Endogene Mikroemboli wurden in einem 40 cm langen Dacron-Segment (4 mm Durchmesser) erzeugt, das während 1 h in den arterio-arteriellen Shunt eingesetzt wurde.

Vor Einsatz des Shunt wurden autologe Plättchen mit ^{111}In-Oxyd [J Clin Invest 1979;64:559–569] markiert und 1,5 mCi intravenös injiziert. Szintigraphische Bilder des Gehirns wurden während des Experiments in posteroanteriorer Position (5-min-Sequenzen) angefertigt. Zusätzlich wurde die Indium-Aktivität einer 4-ml-Blutprobe (Blutstandard) bestimmt. Die Plättchenzahl (markiert und unmarkiert) wurde für jede Hemisphäre nach einer vorbeschriebenen Methode [Stroke, im Druck] bestimmt. Die embolisierten Plättchenpartikeln wurden mit einer kontinuierlichen transkraniellen Doppler-Sonographie erfaßt. Nach Beendigung des Experiments wurde bei 2 Tieren der neurologische Status unter Benutzung einer speziellen Skala nach 1, 12 und 24 h bestimmt. Bei den anderen Tieren wurden die Hirne lichtmikroskopisch untersucht. Thrombozyten, Leukozyten, Fibrinogen, aktivierte partielle Thromboplastinzeit, Fibrinopeptid A, β-Thromboglobulin und Plättchenfaktor 4 wurden vor und 1, 12 und 24 h nach Einsetzen des Dacron-Segments bestimmt.

Unmittelbar nach Eröffnung der Blutzirkulation durch das thrombogene Dacron-Segment registrierte der transkranielle Doppler einen kontinuierlichen Strom von Mikroembolien in der A. carotis interna. Gleichzeitig konnte eine Akkumulation von ^{111}In-markierten Plättchen in der ipsilateralen Hemisphäre erfaßt werden. Der durchschnittliche hemisphärische Basiswert stieg nach 20 min von $0,36 \pm 0,11 \times 10^9$ Plättchen auf ein Maximum von $3,2 \pm 11 \times 10^9$ Plättchen (p < 0,001). Nach 40 min fiel die Zahl der Plättchen auf $1,3 \pm 0,4 \times 10^9$, obwohl das thrombogene Dacron-Segment noch immer als Emboliequelle diente. Nach Entfernung des Dacron-Segments kam es zu einem raschen Abfall der Plättchenzahl aus der zerebralen Zirkulation mit Erreichen des Basiswertes von $0,48 \pm 0,13 \times 10^9$ nach 60 min. In der kontralateralen Hemisphäre fanden sich keine Veränderungen der Plättchenaktivität. Hämatokrit, Leukozytenzahl und Fibrinogengehalt blieben während des Experiments konstant. Die Plättchenzahl im peripheren Blut fiel infolge des Plättchenverbrauchs im Dacron-Segment während der 1. h um 25% von $331\,000 \pm 57\,900$ auf $247\,000 \pm 45\,600$. Die Thrombosemarker im peripheren Blut stiegen alle während der 1. h nach Einsatz des thrombogenen Dacron-Segments an.

Die Werte für β-Thromboglobulin betrugen vor und 60 und 120 min nach Einsatz der Dacron-Prothese $6,9 \pm 1,7$, $127,0 \pm 51,6$ und $33,3 \pm 12,1$ ng/ml; die Werte für Plättchenfaktor 4 waren 7,3 ± 0,6, 54,0 ± 3,9 und 10,8 ± 4,0 ng/ml; für Fibrinopeptid A betrugen sie 3,4 ± 1,6, 32,1 ± 2,8 und 2,3 ± 1,2 nmol/ml; die aktivierte partielle Thromboplastinzeit war 53,9 ± 21,6, 86,2 ± 12,4 und 70,5 ± 2,3 s.

Nach Erwachen aus der Narkose zeigten die beiden Tiere eine milde kontralaterale Hemiparese einschließlich der Gesichtsmuskulatur, wobei sich der neurologische Score von 100 auf 54 bzw. 35 verringert hatte. 12 h später waren die neurologischen Funktionen und auch das Verhalten der Affen wieder normal. Die neuropathologische Untersuchung der druckperfundierten Gehirne zeigte normale Gefäße und, mit Ausnahme eines einzigen Thrombus in einem meningealen Gefäß, keine Hinweise auf Gefäßverschlüsse.

Die hier vorgestellte Untersuchung unterscheidet sich von akuten Verschluß- oder Embolisationsmodellen dadurch, daß durch die Erzeugung von endogenen Plättchenembolien die Interaktionen der Gefäßwand mit Plättchenembolien untersucht werden kann. Es kann nicht nur die Menge der Emboli szintigraphisch quantifiziert und mit dem transkraniellen Doppler erfaßt werden, sondern auch deren Elimination aus der betroffenen Hemisphäre. Es zeigt sich zusätzlich, daß Thrombosemarker im peripheren Blut reagieren und z. B. einen Plättchenverbrauch erkennen lassen. Insgesamt ist das experimentelle Modell gut geeignet, die Pathophysiologie plättchenembolischer Insulte und therapeutische Interventionsmöglichkeiten zu untersuchen.

References

1   Millikan CH, McDowell F, Easton JD: Stroke. Philadelphia, Lea & Febiger, 1987, pp 48–52.
2   Cunning AJ, Pickering GW, Robb-Smith AHT, Russel RR: Mural thrombus of the internal carotid artery and subsequent embolism. Q J Med 1964;33:155–195.
3   Cerebral Embolism Task Force: Cardiogenic brain embolism. Arch Neurol 1986;43:71–84.
4   Migaki G, Casey HW: Animal models of thrombosis and hemorrhagic diseases. Department of Health Eduction and Welfare, Public Health Service, National Institute of Health, Bethesda, pp 5–65 (NIH Publ. No 76-982).
5   Hampton JW, Mathews C: Similarities between baboons and human blood clotting. J Appl Physiol 1966;21:1713–1716.
6   Todd ME, McDevitt EL, Goldsmith EI: Blood-clotting mechanisms of nonhuman primates: Choice of the baboon model to simulate man. J Med Primatol 1972;1:132–141.
7   Harker LA, Hanson SR: Experimental arterial thromboembolism in baboons: Mechanism, quantitation and pharmacologic prevention. J Clin Invest 1979;64:559–569.
8   Kessler CH, Kelly AB, Suggs WD, Weissman JD, Epstein CM, Hanson SR, Harker LA: Induction of transient neurologic dysfunction in baboons by platelet microemboli. Stroke, in press.
9   Spetzler RF, Selman WR, Weinstein P, Townsend J, Mehdorn M, Telles D, Crumrine RC, Macko R: Chronic reversible cerebral ischemia: Evaluation of a new baboon model: Neurosurgery 1980;7:257–261.
10 Del Zoppo GJ, Copeland BR, Harker LA, Waltz TA, Zyroff J, Hanson SR, Battenberger E: Experimental acute thrombotic stroke in baboons. Stroke 1986;17:1254–1265.

11 Symon L: Experimental model of stroke in the baboon. Adv Neurol 1975;10:199–212.
12 Schneider PA, Kotze HF, du Heynes PA, Hanson SR: Thromboembolic potential of synthetic vascular grafts in baboons. J Vasc Surg 1989;10:75–82.
13 Hanson SR, Harker LA, Ratner BD, Hoffman AS: In vivo evaluation of artificial surfaces with a nonhuman primate model arterial thrombosis. J Lab Clin Med 1980;95:289–304.
14 Moncada S: Biological importance of prostacyclin. Br J Pharmacol 1982;76:3–31.
15 Foerstmann U, Warmuth G, Dudel C, Alheid U: Formation, functions and importance of endothelium derived relaxing factor and prostaglandins in the microcirculation. Z Kardiol 1989;78(suppl):85–91.

Prof. Dr. C. M. Kessler
Klinik für Neurologie und Psychiatrie
Ernst-Moritz-Arndt-Universität Greifswald
Ellernholzstraße 1/2
D-17489 Greifswald (FRG)

Dorndorf W, Marx P (eds): Stroke Prevention.
Basel, Karger, 1994, pp 53–66

Hemorheological Risk Factors for Ischemic Stroke

A. Haass

Department of Neurology, University of the Saarland, Homburg/Saar, FRG

Hematocrit as a Risk Factor for Stroke

The high incidence of vascular events in polycythemia vera is well known. The number of vascular occlusive episodes correlates directly with the hematocrit (Hct) range and interestingly does not with platelet counts [34]. Cerebrovascular complications are the most frequent arterial events and they are about four times more frequent than coronary complications pointing to different hemorheological pathomechanisms in cerebral and coronary vessels. Venesection can still be an effective treatment to reduce cerebrovascular events [1].

An Hct value below 0.45 was recommended because it reduced the instance of vascular death to a fairly normal degree [31]. Furthermore, Willison et al. [47] investigated the effect of high and normal Hct values on cerebral function by objective psychological 'alertness' tests. Patients selected by a routine hematological investigation with Hct values above 0.46 showed an impaired performance. The reduction of the Hct to high normal or marginally elevated values by venesection normalized the speed and accuracy of performance and induced an increase of cerebral blood flow (CBF) which correlated with improvement in alertness. Thus for an optimum cerebral function a high CBF is more important than a high oxygen-carrying capacity due to a high Hct.

The early results of the epidemiological Framingham Study were less unequivocal [19] (table 1). High normal or greater Hct values doubled the stroke risk in women (Hb > 14 g/l) and in men (Hb > 15 g/l). Furthermore, Hct was the fourth risk factor after blood pressure, coronary heart disease

Table 1. High Hct as a risk factor for stroke

Study	Risk factor
Framingham study, 1972 [19]	weak risk factor
Toghi et al., 1978 [42]	independent risk factor
Walker et al., 1981 [44]	Hct ↑ risk factor
	Hct ↓ weak risk factor
Harrison et al., 1982 [17]	dependent and independent risk factor
Kiyohara et al., 1986 [22]	dependent risk factor
Koudstaal et al., 1992 [24]	independent risk factor
(n = 3,150)	> 45%, hazard ratio 1.6–1.7
UK-TIA trial, Harrison, 1989 [15]	independent risk factor

and heart frequency [21]. But it was associated to blood pressure and cigarette smoking and seemed to be only a weak independent risk factor.

In the study of Kiyohara et al. [22], Hct was a risk factor for stroke, which was dependent on several additional risk factors including blood pressure and smoking. Toghi et al. [42] and Harrison et al. [17], however, demonstrated that an elevated Hct was a risk factor for stroke and TIA which was dependent as well as independent of hypertension and smoking habit. On the other hand, not contrary to these results, two studies not only confirmed a high Hct as a risk factor, but also under special conditions a very low one, because the latter might well be a consequence of coexisting illness [22, 44].

In respect to the risk of a high Hct, two new investigations now allow a clear conclusion. Recently, in a well-designed multicentre study of 3,150 patients with TIAs or minor stroke, Koudstaal et al. [24] performed multivariate analyses on variables for stroke and confirmed an Hct value of above 0.45 as an independent risk factor for subsequent stroke. Interestingly, this was not the case for vascular death and myocardial infarction, additionally indicating the different hemorheological risks in coronary and cerebral vascular diseases. Furthermore, the authors could predict the hazard ratio, which was 1.6–1.7 and meant that the risk of a high Hct was higher than of a previous minor stroke and lower than of diabetes mellitus for example. The same held true for the UK-TIA trial [15]. Thus from investigations of more than 5,000 patients we can now conclude that an Hct value above 0.45 is a significant risk factor. Interestingly, there is a

Table 2. High Hct and stroke etiologies

Study	Stroke etiology		
Pearce et al., 1983 [33]	polycythemia	→	lacunes
Toghi et al., 1978 [42]	high Hct	→	lacunes
LaRue et al., 1987 [26]	high Hct + hypertension	→	lacunes
Harrison et al., 1981 [16]	high Hct	→	carotid occlusion
Bogousslavski et al., 1986 [2]	high Hct + hypertension + smoking	↓	watershed infarcts carotid occlusion

therapeutic link between a high Hct and antiplatelet therapy. The UK-TIA trial showed that the patients of the placebo group had a stroke risk which was dependent on the Hct value, whereas the risk of the ASA-treated patients was independent of the Hct value. The same risk reduction was seen in the EC-IC bypass study [43], in which all patients were on aspirin. Thus two clinical trials demonstrate that the increased stroke risk of a high Hct is counteracted by ASA therapy. In contrast to the opinion of Back and von Kummer [48], there is no doubt that an increased Hct is a significant risk factor for stroke. Furthermore, the UK-TIA bypass study and the EC-IC study showed that an elevated Hct is an indication for an ASA therapy, and that this therapy is able to normalize the increased stroke risk.

High Hct and the Relation to Stroke Etiologies

A further question is if high Hct values induce specific stroke subtypes (table 2). In accordance to our own observations, Pearce et al. [33] described in case reports the association of lacunar stroke and high Hct. Toghi et al. [42] and LaRue et al. [26] observed more lacunar infarcts than thrombotic or embolic strokes in patients with high Hct. The latter authors could not exclude hypertension as a coexisting factor, which is not surprising, since a high Hct and hypertension are independent but also dependent risk factors. In conclusion, a high Hct contributes to stroke subtypes typical of cerebral microcirculation disturbances.

On the other hand, there are indications that a high Hct also increases the risk for strokes in large vessel diseases. Harrison et al. [16] described that independently of the severity of atheromatous vessel wall changes, carotid occlusion occurred more often among patients with Hct value above 0.50. This was confirmed by the investigations of Bogousslavski et al. [2] who also found high Hct values, especially in patients with internal carotid artery occlusion. Additionally, they described that the occurrence of watershed infarcts was combined surprisingly frequently with an elevated Hct. They concluded that an 'elevated hematocrit increases the risk of infarction, probably by increasing blood viscosity'. Both investigations underline the interaction between hemodynamic mechanisms and hemorheology. Whereas a normal hemodynamic situation may compensate in a certain degree the risk of pathological hemorheological factors, an impaired hemodynamic state, i. e. heart disease with decreased cardiac output, acute lowering of the blood pressure or hemodynamically significant stenosis, increases the risk of hemorheological factors. In macro-circulation disturbances a high Hct especially promotes carotid occlusion and increases the risk of watershed infarcts in patients with carotid occlusion or tight stenosis.

In conclusion, a high Hct is a risk factor for micro- as well as macro-circulation disturbances and should induce prophylactic therapeutic consequences like ASA medication or hemodilution.

Hct and Acute Stroke

There are also indications that an elevated Hct promotes a more unfavorable prognosis of an acute stroke (table 3). The relation between a raised Hct and hospital mortality was examined by Lowe et al. [28]. A very high Hct of 0.50 or above on admission was found in 11% of all patients. The authors excluded dehydration as a main reason for this observation. The significance of a high Hct was especially demonstrated by the high mortality rate of this group, which was more than doubled compared to patients with a lower Hct of 0.40–0.49. These observations were confirmed by Culicchia et al. [4] studying 742 patients, while Ozaita et al. [32] studying only 131 strokes did not agree. These observations are also in accordance with CCT investigations in stroke patients [16] with stroke models in animals [35] and SPECT results in human infarcts [38]. The size of the infarcts of patients and of the gerbil stroke model were shown to be related: the higher the Hct value the larger the size. The SPECT investigations demonstrated that a high Hct in the ischemic region led to a poor clinical outcome for the patients.

The possible mechanisms of the adverse effects of a high Hct include the promotion of the formation of thrombi and the slowing of CBF by the autoregulation and by the increased blood viscosity. They are also the rationale of hemodilution since a high CBF induced by a low Hct seems to be more important for a good clinical prognosis in stroke patients than a high oxygen-carrying capacity due to a high Hct. But in order to understand the contradictory clinical results of hemodilution trials it is necessary to distinguish between the different effects of a hyper-, iso- and hypovolemic hemodilution on cardiac output and on CBF in normal subjects and in patients with an impaired autoregulation in the stroke area. Under normal conditions hemodilution increases CBF because cerebral autoregulation induces compensatory vasodilatation due to deficiency of oxygen delivery. Under these conditions cardiac output and blood pressure do not change CBF due to the intact autoregulation and the Hct has a low effect in the microcirculation. But in the penumbra of stroke the autoregulation is disturbed and therefore coupling of CBF to oxygen content of the tissue is interrupted and the perfusion passively follows the blood pressure and cardiac output. Furthermore, blood viscosity may play a major role under the conditions of an impaired perfusion.

Thus it is of special importance if the well-known increase of CBF under hemodilution is due to a decrease in viscosity and if hyper- and isovolemic hemodilution have different effects on cardiac output.

Recently, Korosue and Heros [23] investigated for the first time if hemodilution in the ischemic penumbra increases CBF by decreasing viscosity or by affecting the vascular autoregulation. They demonstrated

Table 3. High Hct and acute stroke

Study	Result

High Hct
  Harrison et al., 1981 [16]
  Pollock et al., 1982 [35]
	increased size of infarct

High Hct
  Lowe et al., 1983 [28]
  Culicchia et al., 1986 [4]
	increased hospital mortality

High cerebral Hct in the ischemic region Sakai et al., 1989 [38]	poor prognosis

that the increase in CBF in the penumbra was due to a decrease in viscosity and not due to a lowered oxygen transport capacity. With respect to the effect of hemodilution on cardiac output, isovolemic hemodilution had no effect and hypovolemic hemodilution decreased cardiac output we showed that hypervolemic hemodilution decreased cardiac output [14]. Thus hemodilution should be performed in a hypervolemic way adjusted to the cardiac capacity according to the study of Strand et al. [40], which demonstrated a much better clinical outcome for the hemodilution group than for the placebo. This was confirmed by several other studies, whereas lowering the Hct and the cardiac output could have a deleterious effect (for details see [14]).

The SPECT investigations of Sakai et al. [38] also showed that the Hct in the macrocirculation is higher than in the microcirculation and that hemodilution reduced to a great extent the large vessel Hct, whereas the reduction in the Hct of the cerebral microcirculation was minimal. The same results were obtained after hyper- and isovolemic hemodilution measuring the Hct in the large vessels and in cutaneous capillaries in man [13, 18]. Thus the reduction of the Hct by hemodilution does not necessarily decrease the oxygen transport capacity if the hemodynamic state is not impaired by excessive blood-letting or delayed infusion of the plasma expander inducing a hypovolemic and not isovolemic hemodilution [30]. Furthermore, it leads to false-negative data using the Hct values of the large vessels before and after hemodilution to calculate the oxygen transport capacity in the microcirculation [13, 39].

Inhibitors of Platelet Function

The platelet functions include the adhesion, shape change, platelet release reaction and platelet aggregation. It is well known that an increased

Table 4. Platelet in acute stroke and stroke prevention

Platelet acute stroke	Stroke prevention
Thrombocythemia	lacunes
	specific therapy + ASA
Secondary prevention	ASA
	ticlopidine
Acute stroke	ASA

spontaneous platelet aggregation and platelet release reaction is associated with a greater stroke risk (table 4). Two recent investigations showed interestingly that it is not the platelet counts but rather a large platelet size that is an independent risk factor for myocardial as well as cerebral infarction [5, 29].

The preventive risk reduction in stroke by antiplatelet therapy using ASA or ticlopidine is generally accepted, but the most effective dosage of ASA is still in discussion. Three reasons are given for preferring a low ASA dosage, i. e. the inhibition of prostacyclin synthesis by high doses, the inhibition of platelet aggregation as well as thromboxane synthesis by low doses and the adverse effects. There is no doubt that only very low doses of ASA (ca. 40 mg/day) are sufficient to inhibit platelet aggregation and thromboxane synthesis, but there exist also several investigations which demonstrate that higher doses of aspirin (ca. 1000 mg/day) are required to inhibit all platelet functions [25, 41]. Furthermore, no trial with a high ASA dose has demonstrated a less favorable result than trials with low ASA doses. Thus the clinical relevance of a simultaneous inhibition of the prostacyclin synthesis is highly overestimated. Therefore a recently published review on this issue 'raises the possibility that high dose might be better than low dose' [7]. With respect to the side effects of ASA, only the incidence of gastrointestinal adverse effects is strongly dose dependent, whereas the incidence of cerebral hemorrhage is not.

The ASA dilemma that in contrast to myocardial infarction a high dose might be more effective in stroke prevention, yet at the same a high dose increases the gastrointestinal complications, could be solved by using an effervescent formulation of ASA. The effervescent tablets had a higher bioavailability. Thus taking a low dose a high ASA blood concentration will be achieved [37]. Furthermore, a well-designed multicenter study investigating 1,266 men showed that 324 mg ASA in an effervescent buffered powder reduced the gastrointestinal symptoms in the range of the placebo group [27]. In consequence, 400–500 mg ASA as an effervescent tablet seems to be the best medication because it attained a platelet inhibition of a higher ASA dose and had a low incidence of gastrointestinal symptoms like a very low ASA dose.

A comparable alternative to ASA is the new platelet inhibitor ticlopidine, which has different mechanisms of action and side effects compared to ASA [12]. Additionally, ASA sheds a new light on acute stroke therapy. Grotta et al. [9] have already asked whether platelet inhibitor therapy lessens the severity of stroke. Reviewing the data of mild, moderate and fatal stroke, the results from 3 out of 4 stroke prevention studies suggest that strokes in treated patients are less severe than those in untreated patients. In consequence, also acute stroke might be an indication for ASA if an intracerebral hematoma is excluded by CCT.

In essential thrombocythemia, thrombotic and hemorrhagic events occur. Strokes are rare and seem to be of a lacunar subtype. In patients with ischemic events platelet inhibitors are indicated.

Plasma Viscosity and Fibrinogen

The plasma viscosity (PV) exerts its rheological effects mainly in the micro- and not in the macrocirculation (table 5). Large molecules and especially fibrinogen are the important determinants. Several studies proved fibrinogen to be a significant dependent but also independent risk factor for stroke [3, 6, 46]. An increase in fibrinogen is strongly associated with the risk factors of blood pressure, LDL cholesterol and smoking habits. The Framingham Study showed that a high normal level compared to a low normal concentration already doubled the stroke risk [20]. A very interesting detail was published in *Lancet* in 1991. In this study the seasonal change of plasma viscosity and fibrinogen was measured and the latter was 23% higher in winter than in summer. This increase is large enough to contribute to the higher stroke risk in winter. Furthermore, it has to be taken into account that especially patients with hypertension taking diuretics develop not only an increase in Hct but also a dramatic elevation in PV [10]. This may be responsible for the higher stroke rate seen in the MAPHY Study, which compared metoprolol with thiazide diuretics [11, 45]. Especially in severe stroke high fibrinogen concentrations are

Table 5. PV and fibrinogen as a risk factor for stroke

PV + fibrinogen
– Dependent + independent risk factor
– Reduces CBF in microcirculation
Therapy: ancrod
plasma exchange
garlic

associated with an increase in β-thromboglobulin indicating that platelet activation is involved as an important coexisting thrombogenic pathomechanism. Furthermore, atherogenesis is promoted by an interaction of fibrinogen with monocytes and macrophages. An increase of PV especially due to an elevated fibrinogen concentration is not only a significant risk factor for stroke but is also an important determinant of the blood flow in microcirculation.

Ringelstein et al. [36] pointed out that a slightly elevated PV reduced CBF and led to a 'preischemic state'. Reduction of the PV from 1.38 to 1.31 mPAS by ancrod already normalized not only the impaired vasomotor reserve, which was decreased by 25%, but improved also the microcirculation, measured in the retinal capillaries, by about 30%. Thus the reduction of PV and fibrinogen could be a therapeutic opportunity in prophylaxis and in the acute treatment of stroke. Unfortunately an effective reduction of the fibrinogen concentration is only possible using invasive methods like ancrod, plasma exchange, or LDL apheresis. The estrogen, 17β-estradiol, inhibits the synthesis of fibrinogen, but the effectiveness of drug treatment as fibrates, ticlopidine and garlic is unclear.

Leukocyte Adhesion, Deformability and Aggregation

The theoretical and experimental background of the adverse effects of leukocyte activities promoting thrombogenesis and no-reflow phenomenon raises increasing interest. The adverse effects include impaired rheological properties which disturb the microcirculation and are components of the no-reflow phenomenon, and include tissue injury by cytotoxic substances. Increased adhesive properties are also seen in acute stroke [8], but therapeutic consequences could not yet be drawn. Thus it seems to be a light at the end of the tunnel that ticlopidine reduces leukocyte platelet aggregation by inhibiting the platelet-activating factor.

Zusammenfassung

Hemorheologische Risikofaktoren des ischämischen Hirninfarktes

Hämatokrit als Risikofaktor. Die erhöhte Rate von Durchblutungsstörungen bei Patienten mit Polyzythämie ist allgemein bekannt und lenkt die Aufmerksamkeit auf die Wertigkeit eines erhöhten Hämatokrits im Hirnkreislauf. Die Zahl der ischämischen Attacken korreliert direkt mit der Höhe des Hämatokrits und interessanterweise nicht mit der Plättchenzahl. Ischämische Durchblutungsstörungen kommen im zerebralen Kreislauf viermal häufiger vor als im koronaren Bereich, was die unterschiedliche Bedeutung hämorheologischer Faktoren für die einzelnen Gefäßprovinzen unterstreicht. Die isovolämische Hämodilution zur Senkung des Hämatokrits auf Werte unter 0,45 verringert die Gefahr zerebraler Durchblutungsstörungen und verbessert die Hirnleistung dieser Patienten [Willison et al., 1980; Berlin, 1986].

Während frühere epidemiologische Untersuchungen die Bedeutung des Hämatokrits als Risikofaktor für den ischämischen Hirninfarkt unterschiedlich klar belegten, haben neueste umfangreiche Untersuchungen in den Niederlanden und Großbritannien an über 5000 Patienten gesichert, daß ein Hämatokrit über 0,45 ein wesentlicher Risikofaktor für zerebrale Durchblutungsstörungen ist. Die Risikorate beträgt 1,6 bis 1,7 und liegt damit beispielsweise höher als die eines vorausgehenden leichten Hirninfarktes und niedriger als die des Diabetes mellitus [Koudstaal et al., 1992]. Ferner kann aus zwei Untersuchungen abgeleitet werden, daß das hämatokritabhängige erhöhte Hirninfarktrisiko durch die Gabe von Azetylsalizsylsäure normalisiert werden kann, was in der medikamentösen Prävention Berücksichtigung finden sollte [Wade et al., 1987; Harrison, 1989)].

Beziehung zwischen erhöhtem Hämatokrit und zerebralen Mikro- bzw. Makrozirkulationsstörungen. Nach einzelnen Untersuchungen führen die Polyzythämia vera und sekundäre Polyglobulie zu zerebralen Mikrozirkulationsstörungen im Sinne von lakunären Infarkten. Ein erhöhter Hämatokrit fördert aber auch bei Makrozirkulationsstörungen die Entwicklung von A.-carotis-interna-Verschlüssen, und zwar unabhängig vom Schweregrad der Atherosklerose [Harrison et al., 1981; Bogousslavski et al., 1986]. Ferner entwickeln Patienten mit einer hochgradigen A.-carotis-interna-Stenose häufiger einen hämodynamischen Grenzzoneninfarkt, wenn ihr Hämatokrit erhöht ist [Bogousslavski et al., 1986]. Diese Beobachtung unterstreicht die pathophysiologische Bedeutung und das Zusammenspiel zwischen beeinträchtigter Hämodynamik durch eine Gefäßstenose und pathologischen hämorheologischen Parametern, wie einem erhöhten Hämatokrit.

Hämatokrit und akuter ischämischer Hirninfarkt. Nach computertomographischen Untersuchungen entwickelt ein Patient einen um so größeren Hirninfarkt, je höher sein Ausgangshämatokrit ist. Ferner geht ein erhöhter Hämatokrit mit einer erhöhten Mortalität während der stationären Behandlung einher. Nach Spect-Untersuchungen ist die Prognose eines Hirninfarktpatienten um so schlechter, je höher der Hämatokrit im Ischämiebereich ist. Es kommt also offensichtlich bei der Behandlung des ischämischen Hirninfarktes weniger auf eine möglichst hohe Zahl sauerstofftransportierender Erythrozyten an als vielmehr auf eine optimale Hirndurchblutung. Diesen Ansatz verfolgt die Hämodilutionsbehandlung, wobei nach den vorliegenden Studien durch eine hyper-, iso- und hypovolämische Hämodilution unterschiedliche klinische Ergebnisse erzielt wurden. Da die Hämodilution die schon häufig primär schlechte Hämodynamik des Hirninfarktpatienten auf keinen Fall durch eine weitere Verringerung des Herzzeitvolumens ungünstig beeinflussen darf, empfiehlt sich eine an die kardiale Belastbarkeit angepaßte hypervolämische Hämodilution mit Senkung des Hämatokrits um 10% und Steigerung des Herzzeitvolumens um ebenfalls 10% [Strand et al., 1984; Haass et al., 1992].

Thrombozytenfunktionshemmer. Als Thrombozytenfunktionshemmer stehen Azetylsalizylsäure und Ticlopidin zur Verfügung. Die optimale ASS-Dosis ist noch umstritten. Während bei kardialen Indikationen Dosierungen um 100 mg sich als wirksam erwiesen, scheinen im zerebralen Durchblutungsbereich höhere Dosen einen besseren Schutz zu gewährleisten [Dyken et al., 1992]. Wegen der dosisabhängigen gastrointestinalen Nebenwirkungen sind aber Dosen von 1000 mg pro Tag schlecht verträglich. Eine Lösung dieser Probleme bietet sich durch die Verwendung von Brausetabletten an, da sie nach einer umfangreichen Studie die gastrointestinalen Beschwerden nahezu auf die Plazeborate reduzieren und aufgrund der höheren Bioverfügbarkeit Dosen von 400 bis 500 mg einer Wirkung von über 1000 mg mikroverkapselter Tabletten entsprechen [Ross-Lee et al., 1982; Lewis et al., 1983; Haass 1991]. Beim Versagen der ASS-Therapie oder Unverträglichkeit steht Ticlopidin als Alternative zur Verfügung.

Plasmaviskosität und Fibrinogenkonzentration. Eine pathologische Plasmaviskosität, insbesondere aufgrund einer erhöhten Fibrinogenkonzentration, ist nach verschiedenen epidemiologischen Untersuchungen ein wesentlicher Risikofaktor für zerebrale Durchblutungsstörungen. Ferner verringert eine erhöhte Plasmaviskosität die Durchblutung in der zerebralen Mikrozirkulation. Eine Senkung der Fibrinogenkonzentration und damit der Plasmaviskosität von 1,38 auf 1,31 mPas verbessert die zerebrale Vasomotorenreserve um 25% und die Mikrozirkulation um 30% [Ringelstein, 1988].

Leukozytenadhäsion, -verformbarkeit und -aggregation. Die Bedeutung der Leukozytenadhäsion, -verformbarkeit und -aggregation für die Entstehung von kardialen und zerebralen Durchblutungsstörungen, insbesondere für das Ausmaß von Reperfusionsschäden, wurde durch verschiedene tierexperimentelle Untersuchungen nachgewiesen, ohne daß sich bisher daraus wesentliche therapeutische Konsequenzen ableiten ließen. Sowohl von der Azetylsalizylsäure als auch vom Ticlopidin sind hemmende Einflüsse auf diese Leukozytenfunktionen beschrieben worden, so daß diese Angriffspunkte auch ein Teil der Wirkungsmechanismen dieser Substanzen sein können.

References

1   Berlin NI: Polycythemia vera: An update. Semin Hematol 1986;23:131.
2   Bogousslavski J, Regli F: Unilateral watershed cerebral infarcts. Neurology 1986;36:373–377.
3   Coull BM, Beamer N, de Garmo P, Sexton G, Nordt F, Knox R, Seaman GVF: Chronic blood hyperviscosity in subjects with acute stroke, transient ischemic attack, and risk factors for stroke. Stroke 1991;22:162–168.
4   Culicchia F, Tatemichi TK, Mohr JP, Hier DB, Price TR, Wolf PA, Kunitz SC: Hematocrit and acute stroke: The NINDS Stroke Data Bank. Neurology 1986;36:139–140.
5   D'Erasmo E, Aliberti G, Celi FS, Romagnoli E, Vecci E, Mazzuoli GF: Platelet count, mean platelet volume and their relation to prognosis in cerebral infarction. J Intern Med 1990;227:11–14.
6   Di Minno G, Mancini M: Measuring plasma fibrinogen to predict stroke and myocardial infarction. Arteriosclerosis 1990;10:1–7.
7   Dyken ML, Barnett HJM, Easton JD, Fields WS, Fuster V, Hachinski V, Norris JW, Sherman DG: Low-dose aspirin and stroke. 'It ain't necessarily so'. Stroke 1992;23:1395–1399.
8   Grau AJ, Berger E, Sung KLP, Schmid-Schönbein GW: Granulocyte adhesion, deformability, and superoxide formation in acute stroke. Stroke 1992;23:33–39.
9   Grotta JC, Lemak NA, Gary H, Fields WS, Vital D: Does platelet antiaggregant therapy lessen the severity of stroke? Neurology 1985;35:632–636.

10 Grotemeyer KH: Aspekte der hämorheologischen Diagnostik bei zerebralen Ischämien. Med Welt 1992;43:37–41.

11 Grotemeyer KH, Schütt H: Hämorheologische Befunde bei Hirninfarktpatienten. Med Welt 1988;39:771–774.

12 Haass A: Aggregationshemmung oder Antikoagulation bei zerebraler Ischämie; in Weber AM (ed): Aggregationshemmung oder Antikoagulation in Innerer Medizin und Neurologie. München, MMV Medizin Verlag, 1991, pp 80–107.

13 Haass A, Jung F: Haemodilution and oxygen transport capacity. J Neurol 1990;237:126.

14 Haass A, Stoll M, Treib J: Hemodilution in cerebral circulatory disturbances. Indications, implementation, additional drug treatment, and alternatives; in Koscielny J, Jung F, Kiesewetter H, Haass A (eds): Hemodilution. New Aspects in the Management of Circulatory Blood Flow. Improvement of Macro- and Microcirculation. Berlin, Springer, 1992, pp. 53–105.

15 Harrison MJG: Influence of haematocrit in the cerebral circulation. Cerebrovasc Brain Metab Rev 1989;1:55–67.

16 Harrison MJG, Pollock S, Kendall BE, Marshall J: Effect of haemotocrit on carotid stenosis and cerebral infarction. Lancet 1981;ii:114–115.

17 Harrison MJG, Pollock S, Thomas D, Marshall J: Haematocrit, hypertension and smoking in patients with transient ischaemic attacks and in age- and sex-matched controls. J Neurol Neurosurg Psychiatry 1982;45:550–551.

18 Jung F, Koscielny J, Mrowietz C, Wolf S, Kiesewetter H, Wenzel E: Einfluß der Hämodilution auf den systemischen und den Kapillarhämatokrit. Infusionstherapie 1990;17:268–275.

19 Kannel WB, Gordon T, Wolf PA, McNamara P: Hemoglobin and the risk of cerebral infarction: The Framingham Study. Stroke 1972;3:409–420.

20 Kannel WB, Wolf PA, Castelli WP, D'Agostino RB: Fibrinogen and risk of cardiovascular disease: The Framingham Study. J Am Med Assoc 1987;258:1183–1186.

21 Kannel WB, Wolf PA, Verter J: Koronare Herzkrankheit und Apoplexie. Gemeinsamkeiten und Zusammenhänge. J Am Med Assoc 1984;3:403–407.

22 Kiyohara Y, Ueda K, Hasuo Y, Fujii I, Yanai T, Wada J, Kawano H, Shikata T, Omae T, Fujishima M: Hematocrit as a risk factor of cerebral infarction: Long-term prospective population survey in a Japanese rural community. Stroke 1986;17:687–692.

23 Korosue K, Heros RC: Mechanism of cerebral blood flow augmentation by hemodilution in rabbits. Stroke 1992;23:1487–1493.

24 Koudstaal PJ, Algra A, van Gijn K, Kappelle LJ, Pop GAM, van Latum JC, van Swieten JC: Predictors of major vascular events in patients with a transient ischemic attack or non-disabling stroke. Abstractband 65. Jahrestagung der Deutschen Gesellschaft für Neurologie. Kurzfassungen der Vorträge und Poster (1992) 45.

25 Krzywanek HJ, Breddin HK: Platelet inhibitors and the prevention of stroke; in Poeck K, Ringelstein EB, Hacke W (eds): New Trends in Diagnosis and Management of Stroke. Berlin, Springer, 1987, pp 89–95.

26 LaRue L, Alter M, Min Lai S, Friday G, Sobel E, Levitt L, McCoy R, Isack T: Acute stroke, hematocrit, and blood pressure. Stroke 1987;18:565–569.

27 Lewis HD, Davis JW, Archibald DG, Steinke WE, Smitherman TC, Doherty JE, Schnaper HW, LeWinter MM, Linares E, Pouget JM, Sabharwal SC, Chesler E,

DeMots H: Protective effects of aspirin against acute myocardial infarction and death in men with unstable angina. N Engl J Med 1983;309:396–403.

28   Lowe GDO, Jaap AJ, Forbes CD: Relation of atrial fibrillation and high haematocrit to mortality in acute stroke. Lancet 1983;i:784–786.

29   Martin JF, Bath PMW, Burr ML: Influence of platelet size on outcome after myocardial infarction. Lancet 1991;338:1409–1411.

30   Mast H, Marx P: Neurological deterioration under isovolemic hemodilution with hydroxyethyl starch in acute cerebral ischemia. Stroke 1991;22:680–683.

31   Messinezy M, Pearson TC, Prochazka A, Wetherley-Mein G: Treatment of primary proliferative polycythaemia by venesection and low dose busulphan: Retrospective study from one centre. Br J Haematol 1985;61:657–666.

32   Ozaita G, Calandre L, Peinado E, Rodriguez-Antiguedad A, Bermejo F: Hematocrit and clinical outcome in acute cerebral infarction. Stroke 1987;18:1166–1168.

33   Pearce JMS, Chandrasekera CP, Ladusans EJ: Lacunar infarcts in polycythaemia with raised packed cell volumes. Br Med J 1983;287:935–936.

34   Pearson TC, Wetherley-Mein G: Vascular occlusive episodes and venous haematocrit in primary proliferative polycythaemia. Lancet 1978;ii:1219–1222.

35   Pollock S, Tsitsopoulos P, Harrison MJG: The effect of haematocrit on cerebral perfusion and clinical status following carotid occlusion in the gerbil. Stroke 1982;13:167–170.

36   Ringelstein EB, Mauckner A, Schneider R, Sturm W, Doering W, Wolf S, Maurin N, Willmes K, Schlenker, Brückmann H, Eschenfelder V: Effects of enzymatic blood defibrination in subcortical arteriosclerotic encephalopathy. J Neurol Neurosurg Psychiatry 1988;51:1051–1057.

37   Ross-Lee LM, Elms MJ, Cham BE, Bochner F, Bunce IH, Eadie MJ: Plasma levels of aspirin following effervescent and enteric coated tablets, and their effect on platelet function. Eur J Clin Pharmacol 1982;23:545–551.

38   Sakai F, Igarashi H, Suzuki S, Tazaki Y: Cerebral blood flow and cerebral hematocrit in patients with cerebral ischemia measured by single-photon emission computed tomography. Acta Neurol Scan 1989;127:9–13.

39   Scharf J, von Kummer R, Back T, Reich H, Machens G, Wilden B: Haemodilution with dextran 40 and hydroxyethyl starch and its effect on cerebral microcirculation. J Neurol 1989;236:164–167.

40   Strand T, Asplund K, Eriksson S, Hägg E, Lithner F, Wester PO: A randomized controlled trial of hemodilution therapy in acute ischemic stroke. Stroke 1984;15:980–989.

41   Toghi H, Konno S, Tamura K, Kimura B, Kawano K: Effects of low-to-high Doses of Aspirin on platelet aggregability and metabolites of thromboxane A_2 and prostacyclin. Stroke 1992;23:1400–1403.

42   Toghi H, Yamanouchi H, Murakami M, Kameyama M: Importance of the hematocrit as a risk factor in cerebral infarction. Stroke 1978;9:369–374.

43   Wade JPH, Taylor DW, Barnett HJM, Hachinsky VC: Hemaglobin concentration and prognosis in symptomatic obstructive cerebrovascular disease. Stroke 1987;18:68–71.

44   Walker AE, Robins M, Weinfeld FD: The National Survey of Stroke. Clinical findings. Stroke 1981;12(suppl I):13–24.

45   Wikstrand J, Warnold I, Olsson G, Tuomilehto J, Elmfeldt D, Berglund G: Primary prevention with metoprolol in patients with hypertension. Mortality results from the MAPHY Study. J Am Med Assoc 1988;259:1976–1982.

46 Wilhelmsen L, Svärdsudd K, Korsan-Bengtsen K, Larsson B, Welin L, Tibblin G: Fi-
    brinogen as a risk factor for stroke and myocardial infarction. N Engl J Med
    1984;311:501–505.
47 Willison JR, Du Boulay GH, Paul EA, Russel RWR, Thomas DJ, Marshall J, Pearson
    TC, Symon L, Wetherley-Mein G: Effect of high haematocrit on alertness. Lancet
    1980;i:846–848.
48 Back T, von Kummer R: Blutverdünnung bei zerebraler Ischämie. DMW 1989;114:
    350–356.

Prof. Dr. A. Haass
Universitätsnervenklinik und Poliklinik – Neurologie
Universität des Saarlandes
Oscar-Orth-Straße
D-66421 Homburg/Saar (FRG)

Dorndorf W, Marx P (eds): Stroke Prevention.
Basel, Karger, 1994, pp 67–75

Do Risk Factors Relate to Stroke Pattern?

Evidence from the Berlin Stroke Data Bank

P. Marx[a], H. Mast[a], Ch. Schumacher[a], R. Ossmann[b], H. Völler[b]

Departments of [a]Neurology and [b]Cardiology, Steglitz University Hospital,
Free University, Berlin, FRG

Large epidemiological studies [1] have well established the concept of risk factors which accelerate the development of atherosclerosis. Thus, particularly hypertension and diabetes mellitus increase both the risk of coronary and cerebrovascular disease and thereby the risk of myocardial infarction and stroke. Although there has been considerable progress in understanding the molecular mechanisms by which risk factors influence the development of degenerative vascular disease, many questions remain unanswered.

There is, for instance, still no answer to the simple question of why hyperlipidemia is much stronger correlated with coronary than with cerebrovascular disease. Likewise, risk factors may have a different impact at different parts of the vascular tree. There is good evidence from pathoanatomical studies [2] that hypertension leads to cerebral hyalinosis and, consequently, to microvascular infarction and/or intracerebral bleeding. Smoking, on the other hand, may be stronger correlated with disease of the large peripheral vessels and perhaps with disease of the carotid arteries.

We therefore addressed the question whether risk factors for microvascular disease, such as hypertension and diabetes mellitus, are associated with stroke patterns believed to be of microvascular origin.

Unfortunately we can give only preliminary data of 177 consecutive patients who came to our hospital during 1991 with the diagnosis of stroke or TIA. All patients underwent thorough neurological and internal medical examination, CT scanning, Doppler sonography of the carotid arteries, and transthoracic echocardiography. In most patients transesophageal echocardiography was performed as well.

Table 1. Basic data

Median age, years	64	Prior TIA or minor stroke	48
Range, years	29–91	Prior major stroke	35

Table 2. Risk factors

	Present	Absent	Unknown
Hypertension	100	70	7
Diabetes mellitus	58	113	6
Hyperlipidemia	71	102	4
Smoking	62	109	6
Hypertension without diabetes	62*		
Diabetes without hypertension	21*		
Hypertension + diabetes	37*		
Neither hypertension nor diabetes	48*		

* Only patients in whom data collection was complete.

Age, gender, severity of stroke, and history of prior TIA and stroke (table 1) were the same as in other stroke data banks [3].

The risk factor distribution is shown in table 2. Hypertension was present in 100 patients compared to 70 normotensives. In 7 patients, history with regard to hypertension was unclear. Diabetes mellitus was found in 58 out of 177 patients, and hyperlipidemia was detected in 72. 62 individuals smoked until inclusion in the study or had stopped smoking within the last 5 years.

Concentrating upon hypertension and diabetes in patients in whom data collection was complete, there were 62 individuals with hypertension without diabetes, 21 patients with diabetes alone, and 37 with both hypertension and diabetes. 48 patients were free of these two risk factors.

Clinical syndromes and CCT patterns (fig. 1) in patients with or without hypertension did not show significant differences. A few patients were already asymptomatic by the time they reached our hospital. There seems to be a slight tendency for lacunar strokes to occur more frequently in hypertensive (34% of hypertensive individuals) than in nonhypertensive

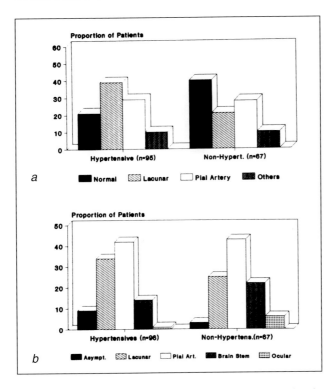

Fig. 1. CCT *(a)* and clinical syndromes *(b)* in all hypertensive and nonhypertensive patients.

(25%) patients. A very similar association emerges if one looks at the CT scans. Lacunes were more often seen in hypertensive (39%) than in nonhypertensive (21%) individuals. Due to the small number of patients, no significant differences emerge from this comparison.

Likewise, the same trend can be seen in diabetic and nondiabetic patients (fig. 2). Lacunar stroke is somewhat more frequent in patients with (42%) than in those without diabetes mellitus (26%). However, neither hypertension nor diabetes had any clear predictive value with regard to lacunar stroke. More than 50% of patients at risk do not present with lacunar syndromes or lacunar stroke.

The data presented so far took in account all patients with a special risk factor and are therefore contaminated by individuals with multiple risk factors. More valid information might be derived from patients with only singular risk factors.

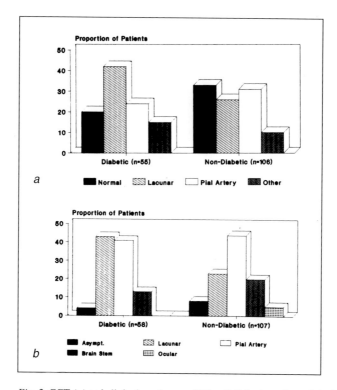

Fig. 2. CCT *(a)* and clinical syndromes *(b)* in all diabetic and nondiabetic patients.

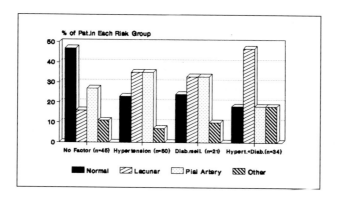

Fig. 3. CCT in patients with different risk factors.

In figure 3 CCT scans of patients with either hypertension or diabetes mellitus or both are compared with individuals having neither hypertension nor diabetes. There were 48 individuals showing none of these risk factors. 62 had hypertension without diabetes and 21 diabetes without hypertension. Finally, there were 37 patients with both hypertension and diabetes.

Again, patients with either hypertension or diabetes mellitus or both presented more often with lacunes than those with no risk factor, and this is particularly true for patients with both hypertension and diabetes mellitus. This result was statistically significant at the 5% level in the chi-square test.

The interpretation of these results is difficult since the concept of lacunar stroke has recently been challenged [4–6] on clinical, radiological, and pathoanatomical grounds. Thus, lacunar syndromes have been documented in patients with nonlacunar CCT pattern. Pathoanatomically some lacunes in the CT scan might not be due to small infarction but rather represent small cavities around a medium-sized intraparenchymal vessel in the basal ganglia ('état crible'), and others might be the remnants of small intracerebral bleedings. According to Ringelstein [5], small borderline infarctions between the striolenticular and insular arteries can easily be mistaken for lacunes. Since we used Ringelstein's definitions, this should not be a major problem in our study.

Most lacunes, however, may be regarded as small infarctions after occlusion of a small intraparenchymal vessel due to microvascular disease. But the possibility, though rare, cannot be excluded that some lacunes may be caused by microembolization from vascular or even cardiac sources.

Although these difficulties cannot be sufficiently resolved, most lacunes may be assumed to originate from microvascular disease, and our data support the hypothesis that both hypertension and diabetes mellitus are particular risk factors for microvascular disease in the brain. The association, however, is week. About two thirds of patients with either hypertension or diabetes mellitus do not have visible lacunes in their CCT scan; and, even in those patients with both hypertension and diabetes, more than 50% are free of lacunes in the CCT. Thus it becomes evident that there must be additional factors or circumstances which influence the development of lacunes. One of these might be the duration of hypertension and/or diabetes mellitus, which has not been sufficiently documented in our data bank so far. But it might also be speculated that inborn susceptibility determinants of the vascular wall itself are of great importance.

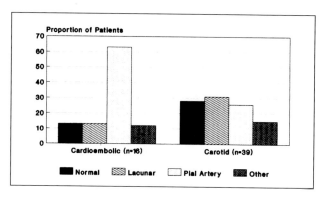

Fig. 4. CCT in presumed cardioembolic and carotid artery stroke.

Hypertension and diabetes are primary risk factors for vascular disease. The increased risk of stroke is only secondary to vascular or cardiac pathology. A look into the literature reveals other types of risk factors: cardiac embolic source or carotid stenosis of more than 50% luminal diameter reduction. In his presentation, Mast [7] has provided strong evidence that by far not all strokes in patients with an accepted source of cardioembolism are really caused by an embolus from the heart.

Therefore, figure 4 does not correlate the CCT pattern of all patients with an accepted cardiac source of embolism but only those in whom clinical evidence strongly indicated cardioembolism as the underlying mechanism. The criteria for allocation to the group 'presumed cardioembolic stroke' were similar to those set up by the NINDS stroke data bank [3] except that we did not include CCT criteria in the selection process. Briefly, only patients with intracavitary thrombi and/or atrial fibrillation were allocated to this group, if there was no carotid stenosis or any other cause of stroke. Carotid stroke was presumed if the patient had an appropriate carotid stenosis but no other source of embolism.

There were only 16 patients who fulfilled the stringent criteria for cardioembolic stroke. In 39 individuals a carotid stenosis was the only detectable cause of stroke.

Pial artery infarction, corresponding to pial artery syndrome, was the most predominant stroke pattern in cardioembolic stroke. About two thirds of patients in this selected group presented with this pattern. This finding is in good agreement with findings of Ringelstein et al. [8].

However, there remain a few patients with lacunar CCT patterns even in this group. Of course, this might be due to concomitant microvascular disease, but lacunes might also be rare sequelae of cardioembolism.

In patients with presumed carotid stroke, lacunar and pial artery patterns were seen in a very similar proportion of CCT scans. This is in good accordance with the assumption that a carotid stenosis may become symptomatic by a variety of mechanisms. First, embolization of thrombotic material may often result in pial artery infarction. But embolization of smaller particles from a carotid plaque could also lead to microinfarction, which might resemble lacunar stroke if located in the basal ganglia. Such a mechanism has been postulated both from clinical and animal studies [for references see 6].

Conclusion

Risk factors for microvascular disease, such as hypertension and diabetes mellitus, are associated with lacunar stroke.

The predictive value of these risk factors is low with regard to microvascular stroke pattern.

Inherited vascular factors probably exert a great influence on the development of degenerative vascular disease.

Cardioembolic stroke is closely associated with pial artery infarction, whereas carotid disease presents with a variety of stroke patterns.

Zusammenfassung

Korrelieren Schlaganfallmuster mit Risikofaktoren?

Pathologisch-anatomisch gibt es Hinweise dafür, daß Hypertonie und Diabetes mellitus neben ihrer Wirksamkeit auf die großen Arterien besonders die Entwicklung einer Mikroangiopathie fördern. Entsprechend wurden lakunäre Infarktmuster im CCT als Hinweis auf eine zerebrale Mikroangiopathie angesehen. Im ersten Teil dieser Studie wird untersucht, ob diese beiden Risikofaktoren mit lakunären Hirninfarktmustern assoziiert sind. Dem werden im zweiten Teil Hirninfarktmuster bei kardialen Emboliequellen und Karotisstenosen gegenübergestellt.

Material und Methoden. In einer prospektiven Studie wurden 177 konsekutiv im Klinikum Steglitz wegen eines TIA oder Hirninfarktes aufgenommene Patienten neben der neurologischen Untersuchung einem CCT, einer Dopplersonographie der Karotiden und einer Echokardiographie (transthorakal und in den meisten Fällen auch transösophageal) unterzogen. Zusätzlich wurden Risikofaktoren, wie Hypertonie und Diabetes mellitus, erfaßt. Die statistische Bearbeitung des Materials erfolgte mittels t-Test und Chi-Quadrat-Test.

Resultate. Alter, Geschlecht, Schwere des Insultes und vorangegangene TIA und Insulte entsprachen denen anderer Schlaganfalldateien. Die Verteilung der wichtigsten Risikofaktoren, Hypertonie und Diabetes mellitus, ist in Tabelle 2 für 168 Patienten mit vollständiger Datenkollektion dargestellt. Lakunen finden sich bei Risikoträgern signifikant (p = 0,05) häufiger als bei Kranken ohne Risikofaktoren. Dies gilt insbesondere für die Kombination von Hypertonie und Diabetes mellitus. Dennoch ist der prädiktive Wert der Risikofaktoren für ein lakunäres Hirninfarktmuster gering: Zwei Drittel der Patienten mit einem und mehr als 50% mit beiden Risikofaktoren weisen keine Lakunen im CCT auf.

Ein Vergleich der CCT-Muster von Kranken mit wahrscheinlich kardioembolischen Insulten (intrakavitäre Thromben oder Vorhofflimmern ohne sonst erkennbare Gefäßstenose oder Embliequelle) und von Patienten mit Karotisstenosen (≥ 50% Lumeneinengung ohne Hinweis auf andere Insultätiologie) zeigt, daß Pialarterien-Infarktmuster bei Patienten mit kardioembolischen Insulten dominieren. Etwa zwei Drittel dieser Kranken weisen das auf eine Embolie hinweisende Infarktmuster auf.

Auffälligerweise läßt sich kein dominierendes Hirninfarktmuster bei Karotisstenosen erkennen: Lakunen, piale und andere Infarktmuster (z. B. Grenzzoneninfarkte) sind ebenso häufig wie Normalbefunde.

Diskussion. Das Konzept, lakunäre Insulte seien ausschließlich Ausdruck einer zerebralen Mikroangiopathie, ist umstritten. Lakunen können zwar Mikroinfarkten infolge eines Verschlusses kleiner striolentikulärer Äste entsprechen, sie können aber auch Reste resorbierter Mikroblutungen sein. Darüber hinaus können sie leicht mit den bei Hypertonus oft erweiterten perivaskulären Hohlräumen («Etat criblé») und mit Grenzzoneninfarkten zwischen den striolentikulären und insularen Arterien verwechselt werden. Handelt es sich um Mikroinfarkte, ist nicht erwiesen, daß diese auf autochthonen Verschlüssen der intraparenchymatösen Gefäße oder auf Mikroembolien, z. B. von der Karotisbifurkation beruhen. Wir fanden eine nur schwache Assoziation von Hypertonie und Diabetes mellitus mit lakunären Infarktmustern. Da die Verlaufsdauer von Hypertonie und Diabetes mellitus und die Kombination mit anderen Risikofaktoren keine Berücksichtigung finden konnten, mag die Risikoexposition nicht immer ausreichend zur Manifestation einer Mikroangiopathie gewesen sein. Darüber hinaus dürften jedoch zusätzliche (genetische?) Faktoren der Gefäßwand den Ablauf des degenerativen Prozesses in der Arterienwand beeinflussen. Die starke Assoziation von Pialarterieninfarktmustern im CCT bei kardialen Embolien steht in guter Übereinstimmung mit Daten von Ringelstein et al. [8]. Die fast gleichmäßige Verteilung der CCT-Muster auf Lakunen, Pialarterien- und Grenzzoneninfarkte bei Karotisstenosen beruht entweder darauf, daß diese Kranken Veränderungen an allen Gefäßabschnitten haben oder darauf, daß Karotisstenosen über unterschiedliche Mechanismen (hämodynamisch bedingte Flußminderung, Embolie atheromatösen und/oder thrombotischen Materials) symptomatisch werden können.

Schlußfolgerungen. Hypertonie und Diabetes mellitus sind mit lakunären Insultmustern assoziiert. Der prädiktive Wert dieser Risikofaktoren für das Hirninfarktmuster ist aber niedrig: Deutlich mehr als 50% der Risikoträger haben keine Lakunen im CCT. Dieser Befund weist darauf hin, daß zusätzliche Faktoren (Dauer der Erkrankung, Kombination mit anderen Risikofaktoren und genetisch determinierte Eigenschaften der Gefäßwand) Einfluß auf die Entwicklung degenerativer Erkrankungen an den unterschiedlichen Gefäßabschnitten haben. Kardioembolische Insulte zeigen eine enge Assoziation mit Pialarterien-Infarktmustern. Karotisinsulte bieten in fast gleicher Verteilung das gesamte Spektrum von Hirninfarktmustern im CCT. Hirninfarktmuster im CCT lassen keine eindeutigen Rückschlüsse auf die Genese des Infarktes zu.

References

1   MacMahon S, Peto R, Cutler J, Collins R, Sorlie P, Neaton J, Abbott R, Godwin J, Dyer A, Stamler J: Blood pressure, stroke, and coronary heart disease. Part 1: Prolonged differences in blood pressure: Prospective observational studies corrected for regression dilution bias. Lancet 1990;335:765–774.

2   Zülch KJ: Die Pathogenese von Massenblutungen und Erweichungen unter besonderer Berücksichtigung klinischer Gesichtspunkte. Acta Neurochir (Wien) 1961(suppl 7):51.

3   Foulkes MA, Wolf PA, Price TR, Mohr JP, Hier DB: The stroke data bank: Design, methods, and baseline characteristics. Stroke 1988;19:547–554.

4   Millican C, Futrell N: The fallacy of the lacune hypothesis. Stroke 1990;21:1251–1257.

5   Ringelstein EB, Weiller C: Hirninfarktmuster im Computertomogramm. Pathophysiologische Konzepte, Validierung und klinische Relevanz. Nervenarzt 1990;61:462–471.

6   Horowitz DR, Tuhrim S, Weinberger JM, Rudolph SH: Mechanisms in lacunar infarction. Stroke 1992;23:325–327.

7   Mast H, Nüssel F, Vogel HP, Heinsius T, Dissmann R, Völler H, Marx P: Cranial Computerized Tomography Stroke Patterns in Patients with Cardiac Sources of Embolism, Extracranial Macroangiopathy or No Extracranial Sources; in Dorndorf W, Marx P (eds): Stroke Prevention. Basel, Karger, 1994, 28–36.

8   Ringelstein EB, Koschorke S, Holling A, Thron A, Lambertz H, Minale C: Computed tomographic patterns of proven embolic brain infarctions. Ann Neurol 1989;26:759–765.

Prof. Dr. P. Marx
Direktor der Abteilung Neurologie
Universitätsklinikum Steglitz
der Freien Universität Berlin
Hindenburgdamm 30
D-12203 Berlin (FRG)

Secondary Prevention in Vascular Disease

Dorndorf W, Marx P (eds): Stroke Prevention.
Basel, Karger, 1994, pp 76–81

Secondary Prevention in Vascular Disease: Assessment of the Risk of Stroke Recurrence

M. G. Hennerici

Department of Neurology, University of Heidelberg, Klinikum Mannheim, FRG

Estimating the stroke risk after a stroke or transient ischemic attack (TIA) represents an important challenge in the attempt to predict the morbidity and mortality associated with cardiovascular diseases. Since cerebral ischemia results from various features of atherothrombotic vascular diseases, e. g. cardiac disease and coronary atherosclerosis, large and small vessel atherosclerosis, disorders of hemostasis, etc., different mechanisms may overlap in repeat events. Thus, coexisting pathomechanisms considerably influence the annual rate of secondary events as does the topography and extent of cerebral ischemia: Bamford et al. [3] suggested that patients with cortical infarction have a higher risk of recurrence (17% in the first year) than those with lacunar subcortical infarctions (9% in the first year).

On the other hand, most of these different pathomechanisms share the involvement of the entire arterial system in the atherosclerotic process. Thus, the risk of fatal and nonfatal myocardial infarction is about the same or greater than the risk of stroke [9], which makes it difficult if not illogical to restrict any analysis of secondary prevention after a first ever stroke only to cerebrovascular events. As a consequence, the efficacy of almost all drugs, which have been studied in large clinical trials, was tested for a statistical estimate of stroke, myocardial infarction and vascular death collectively. Thus, little if any data is available for the prediction of the risk/benefit ratio of any form of management such as medical or surgical treatment of secondary stroke in particular [6].

Another often underestimated important limitation for the prediction of recurrent stroke in a population results from serious referral bias. The risk of stroke is lower in patients refferred to a hospital [7] probably because of different referral habits such as excluding elderly patients with a severe first stroke and preferentially admitting those with a lower mean age and still active mechanisms more likely to be treated effectively, etc. Thus, patients with high-degree carotid stenosis and recent TIAs or mild strokes have clearly been shown to benefit from carotid endarterectomy [12] versus medical treatment whereas those with small carotid plaques may deteriorate from carotid surgery due to the smaller annual rate of spontaneously occurring secondary events [5].

In a recent study, Hankey et al. [7] reported a 4.5% annual death rate and a 6.6% annual stroke rate (first year) and 3.4% (second to fifth year) respectively in patients with TIAs. They are supposed to have a similar prognosis as patients with mild ischemic stroke due to the arbitrary 24-hour limit for the definition of TIA rather than to the activity of different pathomechanisms. This is further supported by a study comparing the risk factors and prognosis for TIAs and minor strokes in a population [4] which demonstrated that the prognosis for TIA and minor stroke did not differ with regard to a subsequent event, whereas patients with minor hemispheric TIA or stroke definitely had a similar but greater risk of subsequent events than those with retinal transient attacks (amaurosis fugax). Furthermore, studies on the natural history of cerebrovascular atherosclerosis have shown that strokes involving brain structures in different vascular territories have a heterogeneous prognosis [3]: In the anterior circulation the morbidity and mortality is high, particularly if cortical rather than subcortical structures are involved, and the chance of clinical recovery is poor. In contrast, patients with infarcts in the posterior circulation have a greater risk of recurrence but a better chance of good functional outcome and a smaller risk for early recurrences but a higher risk for late recurrences. Subcortical infarcts in the territory of small vessels have a yet undetermined prognosis. Arboix et al. [2] favored a prognosis similar to TIA (6.5% annual recurrence rate), which was even smaller than in the series of Bamford et al. [3]. Sacco et al. [13] confirmed these differences in recurrence rates according to the type of stroke: the overall rate at 30 days was 3.3% in more than a thousand patients studied in a Stroke Data Bank with greatest risk of recurrence in patients with atherothrombotic infarcts (7.9%) and least for lacunar infarcts (2.2%).

Risk Reduction and General Strategies

Although reduction of risk factors such as hypertension, diabetes, cigarette smoking, etc., seem to influence prognosis in patients with atherosclerosis, no data are available to support the benefit of such strategies with regard to recurrent strokes. Furthermore, although regression of atherosclerosis has definitely been established to occur pending risk factor reduction [10], this seems to be only true for the initial stages of atherosclerosis rather than for advanced complicated lesions [11].

Medical Treatment – Antiplatelet Drugs

A series of prospective randomized multicenter trials have been conducted to establish the benefit of antiplatelet drugs for secondary prevention of cerebrovascular events. Meta-analysis reports of the Antiplatelet Trialists' Collaboration [1] showed that with regard to combined outcome a 22% overall risk reduction for vascular events (stroke, myocardial infarction and vascular death) occurs. The relative risk reduction for stroke amounts to 30%, for stroke and death 22% and for vascular mortality 15%. The Ticlopidine Aspirin Study [8], which showed a 42% risk reduction for stroke and death and a 47% risk reduction for stroke morbidity and mortality, demonstrated the superiority of ticlopidine over aspirin, and the results of the Canadian-American Ticlopidine Study investigating ticlopidine to placebo in patients with completed major strokes, furthermore, provided evidence that ticlopidine reduced the risk of thromboembolic events by 30% [6]. Unfortunately, neither the mechanisms nor the types of strokes have been addressed in any of these large-scale clinical trials, which increases the difficulty to separate high-risk from low-risk patients.

Surgical Treatment – Carotid Endarterectomy

The North American Symptomatic Carotid Endarterectomy Trial (NASCET) and the European Carotid Surgery Trials (ECST) both being published in 1991 provided evidence for the benefit of carotid surgery in patients with a recent TIA or mild stroke in the territory of a severely obstructed carotid stenosis (> 70% lumen narrowing) although this procedure carries a significant risk (7.5% in ECST and 5.8% in NASCET). Patients were highly selected as were vascular surgeons, and disagreement still exists about the definition of 70% stenosis: probably due to different criteria, the ECST overestimated the degree of stenosis and included more patients with moderate rather than severe stenosis, thus resulting in a less significant difference between the operated and the nonoperated population. Patients with mild stenosis (< 30%) did not benefit from surgery according to the ECST trial whatever the characteristics of the small carotid plaques were (ulcerative or nonulcerative plaques). Patients with moderate stenosis are still under investigation in both trials but are less likely to benefit from surgery as with all those patients with asymptomatic carotid lesions whatever the degree of stenosis and the involvement of different vessels might be [9].

Zusammenfassung

Sekundärprävention bei vaskulären Erkrankungen: Risikovorhersagen für Rezidivinsulte

Die Bestimmung des Rezidivrisikos nach einem Schlaganfall oder nach einem vorübergehenden ischämischen Insult ist ein wichtiger Teilaspekt beim Versuch einer Vorhersage von Morbidität und Mortalität bei kardiovaskulären Erkrankungen. Da zerebrale Ischämien auf unterschiedliche Manifestationen atherothrombotischer Gefäßerkrankungen zurückgehen, wie z. B. kardiale Erkrankungen, Koronarsklerose, Arteriosklerose großer und kleiner Gefäße, Hämostasestörungen usw., können sich unterschiedliche Mechanismen bei Insultrezidiven überlappen. Es wurde darauf hingewiesen [Lancet 1991;337:1521–1526], daß Patienten mit kortikalen Infarkten eine höhere Rezidivrate (17% im 1. Jahr) haben als solche mit lakunären subkortikalen Infarkten (9% im 1. Jahr).

Eine zusätzliche Schwierigkeit der Vorhersage resultiert daraus, daß die verschiedenen *Pathomechanismen* das gesamte arterielle System beeinflussen. So ist das Risiko tödlicher und nichttödlicher Myokardinfarkte gleich groß oder sogar größer als das Schlaganfallrisiko [Brain 1987;110:777]. Es ist daher schwierig, Analysen der Sekundärprävention nach einem ersten ischämischen Insult nur auf zerebrovaskuläre Ereignisse zu beschränken. Die großen klinischen Untersuchungen über die Wirksamkeit von Medikamenten wurden daher meist in bezug auf Schlaganfälle, Myokardinfarkte und vaskulären Tod kollektiv und nicht allein für die Schlaganfallprävention durchgeführt.

Auch die *Patientenrekrutierung* hat Einfluß auf die Schlaganfallerwartung im weiteren Verlauf. So ist das Schlaganfallrisiko bei Krankenhauspatienten niedriger als in einer Gesamtpopulation [J Neurol Neurosurg Psychiatry 1991;54:793–802], was wahrscheinlich daran liegt, daß besonders alte Patienten mit einem schweren Schlaganfall nicht in Krankenhäuser eingewiesen werden, während jüngere Patienten mit höherer Wahrscheinlichkeit behandelt werden können. In dieser Studie wurden darüber hinaus eine Sterblichkeitsrate von 4,5% und eine Schlaganfallrate von 6,6% im 1. Jahr sowie eine Schlaganfallrate von 3,4%/Jahr im 2.–5. Jahr bei Patienten mit vorübergehenden ischämischen Attacken berichtet. In einer gemeindebezogenen Untersuchung [Stroke 1990;21:848–853] war die Prognose von vorübergehenden ischämischen Attacken und leichten Schlaganfällen in bezug auf Rezidivinsulte nicht unterschiedlich. Patienten mit hemispärischen ischämischen Attacken oder Schlaganfällen hatten eine größere Rezidivrate als solche mit Amaurosis fugax.

Außerdem wurde, wie oben erwähnt [Lancet 1991;337:1521–1526], gezeigt, daß Schlaganfälle in unterschiedlichen Hirnstrukturen bzw. *Gefäßterritorien* eine unterschiedliche Prognose haben: Insulte der vorderen Zirkulation haben eine relativ hohe bleibende Morbidität und Mortalität, besonders wenn kortikale im Vergleich zu subkortikalen Strukturen involviert sind. Im Gegensatz dazu haben Patienten mit Infarkten in der hinteren Zirkulation zwar eine höhere Rezidivrate, aber eine bessere Aussicht auf gute funktionelle Restitution. Subkortikale Infarkte im Versorgungsgebiet der kleinen Gefäße haben eine noch nicht eindeutig bestimmte Prognose. In der Literatur [Stroke 1990;21:842–847] wurde eine ähnliche Prognose wie nach vorübergehenden ischämischen Attacken (6,5% jährliche Rezidivrate) beschrieben. Andere Autoren [Stroke 1989;20:983–989] fanden in der Stroke Data Bank eine Gesamtrezidivrate innerhalb von 30 Tagen von 3,3% bei mehr als 1000 Patienten. Das Rezidivrisiko war bei Patienten mit arteriothrombotischen Infarkten mit 7,9% am höchsten, bei solchen mit lakunären Infarkten mit 2,2% am niedrigsten.

Obwohl die *Reduktion von Risikofaktoren*, wie Hypertonie, Diabetes mellitus, Zigarettenrauchen usw., die Prognose von Patienten mit Arteriosklerose zu beeinflussen scheint, liegen keine Daten vor, die den Nutzen solcher Strategien bei der Schlaganfallreduktion belegen. Darüber hinaus scheint eine Regression der Arteriosklerose durch Reduktion der Risikofaktoren im Frühstadium häufiger vorzukommen als bei fortgeschrittener Erkrankung und komplizierten Läsionen [Cerebrovasc Dis 1991;1:142–148].

Eine Reihe prospektiver, randomisierter, multizentrischer Untersuchungen haben eine 22%ige Reduktion des Gesamtrisikos für vaskuläre Erkrankungen (Schlaganfall, Myokardinfarkt und Gefäßtod) unter Azetylsalizylsäure aufgezeigt. Die relative Risikoreduktion für Schlaganfälle betrug 30%, für Schlaganfall und Tod 22% und für Gefäßsterblichkeit 15% [Br Med J 1988;296:320–331]. Die Ticlopidin-Aspirin-Untersuchung [N Engl J Med 1989;321:501–507] wies eine 47%ige Risikoreduktion für Schlaganfallmorbidität und -mortalität nach. Ticlopidin war wirksamer als Aspirin. Die kanadisch-amerikanische Ticlopidin-Studie [Stroke 1988;19:1203–1210] ergab im Vergleich zu Plazebo eine Reduktion thromboembolischer Ereignisse um 30%. Unglücklicherweise sind bei all diesen Untersuchungen die Schlaganfalluntertypen nicht differenziert worden.

NASCET [N Engl J Med 1991;325:445–453] und ECST [Lancet 1991;337:1235–1243] haben gezeigt, daß Patienten mit jüngst durchgemachten vorübergehenden ischämischen Attacken oder leichten Schlaganfällen im Gebiet einer isolierten und hochgradig stenosierten Karotisstenose von einer Karotisendarteriektomie profitieren, obwohl ein signifikantes perioperatives Risiko (7,5% im ECST und 5,8% im NASCET) besteht. Hierbei ist zu bedenken, daß die Patienten ebenso wie die Gefäßchirurgen einer strikten Selektion unterlagen und daß die Definition einer > 70%igen Stenose bei beiden Untersuchungen differierte. Patienten mit leichten Stenosen (< 30%) profitierten nicht von der Karotisendarteriektomie. Die Situation bei Patienten mit mittelgradigen Stenosen ist bisher nicht klar, so daß die Untersuchungen fortgesetzt werden. Wahrscheinlich werden sie weniger von einer Endarteriektomie profitieren als solche mit hochgradigen Stenosen.

References

1   Antiplatelet Trialists' Collaboration: Secondary prevention of vascular disease by pro-
    longed antiplatelet treatment. Br Med J 1988;296:320–331.
2   Arboix A, Martí-Vilalta JL, Garcia JH: Clinical study of 227 patients with lacunar
    infarcts. Stroke 1990;21:842–847.
3   Bamford J, Sandercock P, Dennis M, Warlow C: Classification and natural history of
    clinically identifiable subtypes of cerebral infarction. Lancet 1991;337:1521–1526.
4   Dennis M, Bamford J, Sandercock P, Warlow C: Prognosis of transient ischemic
    attacks in the Oxfordshire Community Stroke Project. Stroke 1990;21:848–853.
5   European Carotid Surgery Trialists' Collaborative Group. MRC European Carotid Sur-
    gery Trial: Interim results for symptomatic patients with severe (70–99%) or with mild
    (1–29%) carotid stenosis. Lancet 1991;337:1235–1243.
6   Gent M, Blakely JA, Easton JD, Ellis DJ, Hachinski VC, Harbison JW, et al.: The
    Canadian American Ticlopidine Study (CATS) in thromboembolic stroke: Design,
    organization and baseline results. Stroke 1988;19:1203–1210.
7   Hankey GJ, Slattery JM, Warlow CP: The prognosis of hospital-referred transient
    ischemic attacks. J Neurol Neurosurg Psychiatry 1991;54:793–802.
8   Hass WK, Easton JD, Adams HP Jr, Pryse-Phillips W, Molony BA, Anderson S,
    Kamm B: A randomized trial comparing ticlopidine hydrochloride with aspirin for the
    prevention of stroke in high-risk patients. N Engl J Med 1989;321:501–507.
9   Hennerici M, Hülsbömer H-B, Hefter H, Lammerts D; Rautenberg W: Natural history
    of asymptomatic extracranial arterial disease. Results of a long-term prospective study.
    Brain 1987;110:777–791.
10 Hennerici M: Regression of atherosclerosis; in Norris JW, Hachinski VC (eds): Preven-
    tion of Stroke. New York, Springer, 1991, pp 49–64.
11 Hennerici M, Steinke W: Carotid plaque developments – Aspects of hemodynamic and
    vessel wall platelet interaction. Cerebrovasc Dis 1991;1:142–148.
12 North American Symptomatic Carotid Endarterectomy Trial Collaborators: Beneficial
    effect of carotid endarterectomy in symptomatic patients with high-grade carotid steno-
    sis. N Engl J Med 1991;325:445–453.
13 Sacco RL, Foulkes MA, Mohr JP, Wolf PA, Hier DB, Price TR: Determinants of early
    recurrence of cerebral infarction. The Stroke Data Bank. Stroke 1989;20:983–989.

Prof. Dr. M. G. Hennerici
Neurologische Klinik am Klinikum Mannheim
Ruprecht-Karls-Universität Heidelberg
Theodor-Kutzer-Ufer
D-68135 Mannheim (FRG)

Dorndorf W, Marx P (eds): Stroke Prevention.
Basel, Karger, 1994, pp 82–90

Can We Compare the Four Main Studies of Secondary Prevention of Ischemic Lesions of the Nervous System (European Stroke Prevention Study, United Kingdom-TIA Study, Canadian-American Ticlopidine Study and Swedish Aspirin Low-Dose Trial)?

A. Lowenthal[a], P. Smets[b]

[a] Medical Research OCMW, Antwerp;
[b] Laboratoire de Statistiques Médicales, Ecole de Santé Publique, ULB, Brussels, Belgium

Introduction

Comparing the different studies of secondary prevention of thromboembolic ischemic lesions of the nervous system by antiaggregating substances is difficult. The antiplatelet trialists (APT) group of Oxford made a basic and very important work by collecting the results of all the studies (published or not), not only for prevention of ischemic lesions of the nervous system, but also for the prevention in the myocardium. Although their conclusions bring useful information and confirm that antiaggregating substances prevent new ischemic lesions, one cannot neglect that studies were associated in their metaanalysis or overview, which had very different inclusion criteria and different numbers of patients, different medications, different doses of a same medication and where the duration of the follow-ups varies and where the endpoints are not the same. For these reasons, we thought that it would be interesting (1) to discuss the methodology of meta-analysis or overview, and (2) to compare from a more clinical point of view the results obtained in the largest studies: the United Kingdom-TIA Aspirin Study, the Canadian-American Ticlopidine Study (CATS), the European Stroke Prevention Study (ESPS-1) and the Swedish

Aspirin Low-Dose Trial (SALT), hoping that such comparison allows to draw practical clinical conclusions. Previous studies as the American-Canadian study and the AICLA were not considered because they recruited less than 1,000 patients.

Results

Critical Evaluation of the Metaanalysis Technique

Clinicians are confronted with clinical trials focusing on similar problems. They must be able to synthesize their results even when they are inconsistent. The meta-analysis tool has been widely advocated to synthesize results from such clinical trials in order to disclose effects that were not obviously shown in each individual trial but might clearly appear when data are appropriately pooled [5]. But, such methodology is muddled by problems related to the interpretation of the results as the data may come from not strictly identical trials. Just as an example of such a danger, consider six clinical trials with independent samples, each comparing in a parallel way a placebo group with a treatment group. Five of them are based on samples of 200 patients per group and the patients in the treatment group received drug X. The sixth trial is based on a sample of 1,000 patients per group and the patients in the treatment group received drugs X and Y in combination. The studied end-point is death within 2 years.

Suppose drug X has no effect and the natural death rate is 25% within 2 years. Suppose Y reduces death rate by half, and does not interact with drug X. Table 1 presents the results as they could be observed (the observed frequencies correspond to the expected frequencies). Of course, the difference between the survival rates in the five first studies is statistically nonsignificant whereas it is statistically highly significant in the sixth study. To process these data in a metaanalysis to test the possible effect of drug X, one pools all the results. The difference between the observed overall death rates is statistically highly significant. A careless interpretation of this metaanalysis leads to the absurd conclusion that drug X is active. Of course, users of metaanalysis are aware of the danger of such careless interpretation, but with less obvious data – where small differences are observed – it becomes less easy to differentiate between appropriate metaanalysis and sheer nonsense as shown in the illustrative example of table 1. So beside metaanalysis, direct comparisons between trials are also useful to be able to synthesize the conclusions of different trials.

Table 1. Simulated results of six clinical trials and their metaanalysis

Treatment	Treated group		Placebo group		Test
	sample size	deaths	sample size	deaths	
X	200	50	200	50	NS
X	200	50	200	50	NS
X	200	50	200	50	NS
X	200	50	200	50	NS
X	200	50	200	50	NS
X and Y	1,000	125	1,000	250	**
Pooled data	2,000	375	2,000	500	**

** p < 0.01.
NS = Not signifikant.

Table 2. Comparison of four studies

Study	Inclusion criteria	End-points	Duration of follow-up (maximum)	Antiaggregating therapy
ESPS-1	TIA, RIND or stroke	stroke + death	2 years	DP 225 mg ASA 990 mg
UK-TIA	TIA or RIND	stroke, myocardial infarction and vascular death	4 years	ASA 300 or 1,200 mg
Ticlopidine	TIA or stroke	stroke, myocardial infarction and vascular death	3 years	ticlopidine 500 mg
SALT	TIA, minor stroke or arterial occlusion	stroke + death	5 years	ASA 75 mg

Direct Comparison of the Results of the Four Main Studies

(A) The *methodology* used allows us to draw our conclusions by comparing results that were published in different papers [2–4, 6–8], or in the overview published by the APT group [1]. We used also the unpublished report of the last meeting of the APT group in Oxford. It was admitted that this report can be used, but not quoted. Some of the mentioned results are only taken out from these publications. Recalculations were only done

Table 3. Comparison of recalculated nonactuarial ESPS results and the published actuarial results (intention to treat analysis on $2 \times 1,250$ patients)

	Number of end-points		Percent end-points		Recalculated RR	Actuarial RR
	DP/ASA	placebo	DP/ASA	placebo		
Global results	190	283	15.2	22.6	32.9 ± 4.8	33.5 ± 5.0
Stroke	114	181	9.1	14.7	38.0 ± 6.1	38.1 ± 7.3
Fatal stroke	22	44	1.8	3.5	50.0 ± 12.9	38.7 ± 20.0
Deaths	108	156	8.6	12.5	30.8 ± 6.8	30.6 ± 8.2
Ischemic deaths	52	83	4.2	6.6	37.3 ± 9.4	34.8 ± 11.4
Myocardial infarction	39	64	3.1	5.1	39.1 ± 10.7	38.9 ± 12.2

from published results. Using always actuarial methods was for evident reasons impossible.

In all these studies, the active arm was compared to a placebo (table 2). For the *United Kingdom study* [6, 7], also the figures published in the overview of the APT group were used [1]. The study included 2,435 patients with a follow-up of sometimes 4 years. The daily regimen was 300 or 1,200 mg acetylsalicylic acid (ASA) or a placebo.

For the *CATS* study only the published figures [4] in intention to treat analysis were used for 1,053 patients with a follow-up of 3 years. 500 mg ticlopidine were prescribed daily or a placebo.

For *ESPS-1* we used the figures published in two papers [2, 3] and the figures published by the APT group [1]. In this 2,500 patient study, with a follow-up of 2 years, we had also the opportunity to compare the actuarial results with the calculations that we did with the published figures. The ESPS [1] patients received t.i.d. 75 mg dipyridamole (DP) and 330 mg ASA or a placebo.

For the *SALT study* the published results [8] were obtained with 1,360 patients followed during a maximum of 5 years and 3 months, receiving either 75 mg ASA or a placebo. Only figures observed in intention to treat analysis were used, although as well for CATS as for ESPS-1, the risk reduction figures are larger in explanatory or efficacy analysis.

All comparisons are based on the risk reduction (RR):

$$RR = \frac{(PC - PT)}{PC}$$

Table 4. Comparison of end-points reduction of four studies: ESPS-1, UK-TIA study, CATS study and SALT study

A. Number of end-points

	ESPS-1 (2 × 1,250 patients)		UK-TIA (1,621 + 814 patients)		CATS (525 + 528 patients)		SALT (676 + 684 patients)	
	DP / ASA	placebo	ASA	placebo	ticlopidine	placebo	ASA	placebo
Stroke + myocardial infarction + vascular death	177	263	354	211	106	134	163	193
Vascular death (after stroke or myocardial infarction) + sudden death + unknown	79	106	180	86	32	41	50	51

B. Percent of end-points and of RR

	ESPS-1 EP, %		RR, %	UK-TIA EP, %		RR, %	CATS EP, %		RR, %	SALT EP, %		RR, %
	DP / ASA	placebo		ASA	placebo		ticlopid.	placebo		ASA	placebo	
Stroke + myocardial infarction + vascular death	14.2	21.0	32.7 ± 6.0	21.8	25.9	15.8 ± 6.4	20.2	25.4	20.4 ± 9.1	24.1	28.2	14.5 ± 7.8
Vascular death (after stroke or myccardial infarction) + sudden death + unknown	6.3	8.5	25.5 ± 10.5	11.1	10.6	5.1 ± 13.0	6.1	7.8	21.5 ± 17.9	7.4	7.5	0.1 ± 19.0

where PT and PC are the proportions of events in the treatment and the control groups, respectively. The correct computation of RR should be based on the estimation of the respective probabilities derived from the survival curves (referred here as the actuarial method). The published results do not permit to take into consideration censored data (lost to follow-up and withdrawn alive). So we used an approximate method where the used proportions are based on the number of events and the number of patients at entry. The proportion of censored data being not too large and the censoring patterns being similar in both groups, the so computed RR might be good approximations of the better estimates derived from the actuarial method (table 3). Each RR is presented in percent with its standard deviation.

(B) We subdivided the *results* that we discuss into two groups:

(1) *We compared the real actuarial results with the recalculated results.* This comparison was only possible for ESPS-1 because here only we had the actuarial figures as we conducted this study (table 3). It is clearly shown that there are no clinical valuable differences between the recalculated RR or the RR following actuarial evaluation.

(2) The second question we tried to answer was to know *how far we can go in the comparison* between the four studies (table 4). It was not possible to compare all the items. Some of the items mentioned are not clearly defined in the published papers, as for instance the difference between new vascular events and the end-points stroke, myocardial infarction and vascular death in ESPS-1 or in the UK-TIA study. The antiaggregating regimen and the duration of the follow-up were not the same in these four studies. Nevertheless, table 4 shows very clearly that in the comparable items the RR is higher for ticlopidine than for ASA alone, but the best figures are observed with the association DP/ASA. For instance, reduction of combined outcome vascular deaths + non-fatal strokes + myocardial infarction is 32.7% with DP/ASA association in ESPS-1, 20.4% with ticlopidine and only 15.8–14.5% with ASA alone.

Discussion

The following conclusions can be drawn from the presented results, and we remind that some results are copied and others recalculated from the published papers:

(A) The proposed *recalculation method* can be useful to compare published material.

(B) From previously published papers it clearly appears that *the antiaggregating therapy can reduce the risk of new vascular events* at the level of the myocardium or of the brain and provides a very clear and very important protection against new vascular lesions. Nevertheless, those papers do not answer two questions: Which antiaggregating substances should be preferentially used? Which dosage is necessary to obtain the best and the less expensive prevention?

(C) ASA in a dosage between 75 and 1,200 mg, although efficient, does not provide the best results, neither for protection of myocardium nor for protection of the brain. Ticlopidine is more efficient than ASA alone, but *the combination DP/ASA is the most efficient* (table 4).

(D) The results of the studies performed until now with antiaggregating substances constitute a very important step forward in the prevention of thrombotic lesions of myocardium and nervous system, but *do not answer the following questions*: (a) Which is the optimal dosage of ASA or DP that should be used? (b) Can we decrease the side effects incidence due to ASA by reducing its dosage? How would this influence the efficacy of the prevention? (c) Can we compensate an eventual loss of efficacy due to a low dosage of ASA by associating it with another antiaggregating agent?

With this in mind, the European Stroke Prevention Study 2 was organized and may give answers to these questions in 1995.

Acknowledgement

We wish to thank Drs J. M. Bertrand-Hardy, A. Goosens, C. Hoeven and S. Schapira for their cooperation in preparing this paper.

Zusammenfassung

Vergleich der vier größten Studien über die Sekundärprophylaxe ischämischer Läsionen des zentralen Nervensystems

Metaanalysen, wie die der Antiplatelet Trialists' Collaboration [Br Med J 1988; 296:320–331], bergen erhebliche methodische Schwierigkeiten in sich, da sie Studien mit unterschiedlichen Einschlußkriterien, Patientenzahlen, Medikamenten sowie unterschiedlichen

Dosierungen eines Medikamentes miteinander vergleichen, wobei auch noch Nachbeobach-
tungszeiten und Endpunkte der Untersuchungen variieren. Die Fallen lassen sich an einem
einfachen Beispiel darstellen: Sechs Studien vergleichen parallel eine Gruppe, die Plazebo
erhielt, mit einer Gruppe, die mit Verum behandelt wurde. Fünf Studien basieren auf je 200
Patienten, die das Medikament X erhielten. Die 6. Studie umfaßt 1000 Patienten, die neben
dem Medikament X auch das Medikament Y erhielten. Nehmen wir an, Medikament X hat
keine Wirkung und die natürliche Sterblichkeitsrate beläuft sich auf 25% in 2 Jahren. Medikament Y reduziert die Sterblichkeit um die Hälfte und interagiert nicht mit Medikament X.
In diesem Fall ergeben die Studien 1–5 keine signifikanten Unterschiede zu Plazebo. Alle
sechs Studien zusammen ergeben jedoch eine signifikante Sterblichkeitsreduktion, die man
natürlich nicht auf Medikament X beziehen darf. Selbstverständlich haben die Autoren der
Metaanalysen derartig leichtsinnige und fahrlässige Fehler vermieden; die prinzipiellen
Schwierigkeiten bleiben jedoch bestehen.

Wir haben daher einen direkten Vergleich von vier besonders großen und bedeutsamen
Studien bevorzugt: 1. die European Stroke Prevention Study [Stroke 1990;21:1122–1130],
2. die Canadian-American Ticlopidine Study [Lancet 1989;i:1215–1220], 3. die UK-TIA
Study [J Neurol Neurosurg Psychiatry 1991;54:1044–1054] und 4. den Swedish Aspirin
Low-Dose Trial [Lancet 1991;338:1345–1349].

Die 3. Studie verglich bei insgesamt 2435 Patienten mit einer Nachbeobachtungszeit
von bis zu 4 Jahren die Wirkung von 300 oder 1200 mg Aspirin mit Plazebo. Die 2. Studie
prüfte 500 mg Ticlopidin gegenüber Plazebo an 1053 Patienten mit einer Nachbeobachtungszeit von 3 Jahren. Die 1. Studie prüfte die Kombination von 225 mg Dipyridamol plus
990 mg Aspirin gegenüber Plazebo an 2500 Patienten mit einer Nachbeobachtungsdauer von
2 Jahren. Die 4. Studie verglich die Wirkung von 75 mg Aspirin bei 1360 Patienten mit einer
maximalen Nachbeobachtungszeit von 5 Jahren und 3 Monaten mit Plazebo. Für alle Untersuchungen wurde die Intention-to-Treat-Analyse benutzt. Die Vergleiche basieren auf der
nach folgender Formel zu berechnenden Risikoreduktion (RR): $RR = (PC - PT) / PC$ (siehe
Text).

PT und PC bezeichnen die Prozentwerte der Endpunktereignisse in der jeweiligen Be-
handlungs- und Kontrollgruppe. Eine Kalkulation der RR auf der Basis der Überlebenskurven war nicht möglich, da die publizierten Resultate dies nicht gestatteten. Es wurde daher
eine approximative Methode angewandt, bei der die Prozentwerte auf der Zahl der Endpunktereignisse und der Patienten bei Studieneintritt basieren. Ein Vergleich der RR aufgrund der
Überlebenskurve und der approximativen Berechnung war nur für die 1. Studie möglich und
zeigte, daß klinisch wichtige Unterschiede der RR durch die beiden unterschiedlichen
Berechnungsarten nicht entstanden. Die Ergebnisse sind in der Tabelle 4 (siehe Text) dargestellt.

Die Resultate zeigen deutlich, daß eine antiaggregierende Therapie bei der Sekundär-
prophylaxe das Risiko neuer vaskulärer Ereignisse reduzieren kann. Es ist aus der erwähnten
Tabelle ebenfalls ersichtlich, daß die größte RR durch die Kombination von Dipyridamol und
Aspirin zu erzielen war.

Zukünftige Untersuchungen, wie die European Stroke Prevention Study 2, sollten folgende Fragen bearbeiten: 1. Welches ist die optimale Dosierung von Dipyridamol und Aspirin? 2. Können Nebenwirkungen von Aspirin durch Dosisanpassungen verringert werden,
und wie beeinflußt dies die Wirksamkeit? 3. Kann eine eventuelle Verminderung der Wirkung von Aspirin in niedriger Dosierung durch Kombination mit anderen antiaggregierenden
Substanzen kompensiert werden?

References

1   Antiplatelet Trialists' Collaboration: Secondary prevention of vascular disease by pro-
    longed antiplatelet treatment. Br Med J 1988;296:320–331.
2   ESPS Group: The European Stroke Prevention Study (ESPS). Principal end-points.
    Lancet 1987;ii:1351–1354.
3   ESPS Group: European Stroke Prevention Study. Stroke 1990;21:1122–1130.
4   Gent M, Easton JD, Hachinski VC, Panak E, Sicurella J, Blakely A, Ellis DJ, Harrison
    JW, Roberts RS, Turpie AGG and the CATS Group: The Canadian-American Ticlopi-
    dine Study (CATS) in Thromboembolic Stroke. Lancet 1989;i:1215–1220.
5   Mann C: Meta-analysis in the breech. Science 1990;249:476–480.
6   UK-TIA Study Group: United Kingdom Transient Ischaemic Attack (UK-TIA) Aspirin
    Trial: Interim results. Br Med 1988;296:316–320.
7   UK-TIA Study Group: The United Kingdom Transient Ischaemic Attack (UK-TIA)
    Aspirin Trial: Final results. J Neurol Neurosurg Psychiatry 1991;54:1044–1054.
8   The SALT Collaborative Group: Swedish Aspirin Low-Dose Trial (SALT) of 75 mg
    aspirin as secondary prophylaxis after cerebrovascular ischaemic events. Lancet
    1991;338:1345–1349.
9   Warlow C: Ticlopidine, a new antithrombotic drug: But is it better than aspirin for
    long-term use? J Neurol Neurosurg Psychiatry 1990;53:185–187.

Dr. A. Lowenthal
106 Jan Van Rijswijcklaan
B-2018 Antwerp (Belgium)

Dorndorf W, Marx P (eds): Stroke Prevention.
Basel, Karger, 1994, pp 91–102

Ticlopidine in the Prevention of Stroke

W. Pryse-Phillips

Department of Neurology, University of Newfoundland, St. John's, Nfld., Canada

Introduction

The reports of Lawrence Craven [1, 2] from his Glendale general practice in the 1950s were ignored for 20 years until Barnett [3] demonstrated that aspirin does indeed reduce the risk of completed stroke following transient ischemic attack (TIA) or minor stroke. Since then, other drugs affecting platelets have been examined for their potency in preventing subsequent strokes. One of these is *ticlopidine*, a thienopyridine derivative which inhibits primary and secondary platelet aggregation in response to ADP, PAF, collagen or thrombin but not to arachidonic acid [4]. It decreases blood viscosity and platelet deposition on atheromatous plaques, enhances platelet disaggregation in normal people and thus increases bleeding times, facilitates red cell deformability and normalizes platelet adhesiveness in diabetic patients. Precisely how it does all this is still undetermined but it seems to act at an early stage in the process of platelet activation.

'Primary' Prevention

Recent trials [5, 6] suggest that, as a primary prevention agent, ASA may *either* double the risk of ICH *or* confer no excess risk at all but it certainly confers protection against myocardial infarction (MI). The risk-benefit equation of trying to prevent MI using therapy which may increase some strokes has yet to be determined.

The Swedish Ticlopidine Multicentre Study [7] was a double-blind placebo-controlled trial designed to determine whether ticlopidine 250 mg twice daily reduces the incidence of MI, stroke and TIAs in 687 patients (76% males) with intermittent claudication studied over 5–7 years or until an end-point was reached. Intention-to-treat analysis showed that in the ticlopidine-treated group, the number of end-points was not significantly lower but that the mortality rate was 29.1% below that in the placebo group (p = 0.015), due to reduced mortality from ischemic heart disease. Ticlopidine was not shown to confer protection in the 'primary' prevention of TIAs nor of ABIs in this study.

'Secondary' Prevention

The four largest trials of antiplatelet drugs in 'secondary' prevention against stroke following TIA, RIND or minor stroke [3, 8–10] all showed a benefit from ASA, which in the Canadian trial offered risk reductions of up to 48% (e. g., for nonfatal stroke and death following TIA in men). Meta-analytic data manipulation indicates that an odds reduction of 22 ± 5% in the risk of subsequent stroke, MI or vascular death was achieved by antiplatelet agents in a composite of all cerebrovascular trials up to 1988 [11]. Put the other way, 73–83% of such events are *not* prevented. Improvement in the event rates has been sought through the use of ticlopidine; two major trials of this agent will be reviewed.

The Ticlopidine-Aspirin Stroke Study (TASS)

In this large trial [12], patients with recent TIA, TMB, RIND or minor stroke were randomly assigned to treatment with either ticlopidine 250 mg twice daily or aspirin 650 mg twice daily and were studied over 5.8 years. The primary end-point was death or nonfatal stroke (thus including fatal strokes as well) and the secondary end-point was the first fatal or nonfatal stroke.

Results

Of the 3,069 eligible patients randomized, 1,529 were assigned to (and 1,518 took) ticlopidine; of the 1,540 assigned to aspirin, 1,527 took it. Men comprised two-thirds of the study population. The average age was 63 ± 9 years (range 39–94 years). Of the qualifying ischemic events, 70% were judged to be in carotid territory, 25% vertebrobasilar. Fifty-two percent of the patients taking ticlopidine and 47% of those taking aspirin stopped treatment before that time.

Using ITT analysis, ticlopidine achieved a 21% (1–36%) reduction in stroke and an 8% (24% to + 12%) reduction in stroke or vascular death when compared to aspirin. Using efficacy analysis (but spanning the whole of the follow-up period), 164 patients on ticlopidine and 220 on aspirin experienced one of the primary outcome events (death from any cause or nonfatal stroke). The cumulative event rates at 12, 24 and 36 months showed risk reductions in favor of ticlopidine, although this reduction diminished over the 3-year period.

Fatal or nonfatal strokes occurred in 111 patients on ticlopidine and in 165 on aspirin, the cumulative event rate showing a significant benefit in favor of ticlopidine (p = 0.011), again more obviously in women.

Subgroup analysis showed that aspirin-treated patients on anti-coagulants or antiplatelet drugs prior to entry into the TASS trial, or with hypertension, diabetes, carotid bruits or elevated creatinine levels had significantly (p ≤ 0.01) more fatal or nonfatal strokes than those without that characteristic. Ticlopidine-treated women, those with hematocrit < 47% and those with abnormal ECG had significantly (p ≤ 0.01) fewer fatal or nonfatal strokes than those without that characteristic. Patients with carotid symptoms treated with aspirin had the highest incidence of subsequent stroke, and those treated with ticlopidine and with vertebroba-silar symptoms had the lowest (p ≤ 0.0003, Wilcoxon and Mantel-Cox). Ticlopidine was more effective than aspirin in preventing subsequent strokes in patients with carotid symptoms but without high-grade stenosis of the carotid arteries, but less effective in those with stenosis of 70% or more (p = 0.009) [13].

Comment

Two reasons may be adduced for the apparent reduction in efficacy of the drugs over the 3 years. First, the risk of stroke is far greater in the first year than in either of the next 2, so there was less room for superior results to be displayed after the first year. Second, those destined to suffer a stroke were likely to do so earlier, so the population in whom risk reduction was being sought was both smaller and progressively less likely to have a stroke anyway. Since the greatest need for prevention against stroke is in the early period after the TIA or other warning, this emphatic early response to ticlopidine is a point in favor of using the drug, accentuating the overall relative superiority of ticlopidine over aspirin as shown in this study.

Although the pathogeneses of TIA and of ABI overlap, the effect of antiplatelet drugs has been examined more often (but shown to be of value almost uniquely) in the case of TIAs. Less than 20% of thromboembolic strokes are preceded by TIAs [14] while after recovery from thromboembolic stroke, the rate of subsequent stroke, MI or vascular death has been reported as nearly 20% at 1 year and about 25% after 2 years [14].

In the ESPS [15], patients with completed stroke comprised some 60% of all entered patients, but the effect of ASA/dipyridamole in preventing different types of cerebrovascular event was not assessed. A Swedish trial of high-dose aspirin following complete stroke did not show that it conferred any benefit [16] but indirect analysis [11] suggested that ASA 300–325 or 900–1,500 mg/day, ASA with dipyridamole, sulfinpyrazone and ticlopidine do *all* reduce the risk of nonfatal stroke and MI (by about 30%) and of vascular death (by $15 \pm 4\%$). The direct analysis will never be done. A study of ticlopidine's effect in the prevention of recurrent stroke was therefore appropriate, and in the absence of evidence of benefit from single studies of other treatments it was possible to employ a placebo control arm.

The Canadian-American Ticlopidine Study (CATS)

In the CATS [17], 1,053 patients with thromboembolic stroke (but not cardioembolic infarcts) were evaluated for a mean of 2 years. The primary end-point for the assessment of efficacy was nonfatal stroke, nonfatal MI and vascular death. Secondary end-points were fatal and nonfatal stroke and deaths from all causes + nonfatal stroke.

Results

1,072 patients were randomized, of whom 19 were ruled truly ineligible. Recurrence of stroke was the most frequent first outcome event. For the primary group of first vascular outcomes among 1,053 patients, there were 118 events in the placebo group over 773 patient-years at risk, an average rate of 15.3% / year. There were 74 events in the ticlopidine group over 683 patient-years at risk, an average rate of 10.8% / year. Ticlopidine thus provided a risk reduction of 30.2% (7.5% to –48.3%; $p = 0.006$) in the incidence of stroke, MI or vascular death (28.1% for males ($p = 0.037$) and 32.4% for females ($p = 0.045$)).

The benefits to ticlopidine were greatest when the outcomes were restricted to vascular events (for the secondary end-point of fatal and nonfatal stroke, the risk reduction was 33.5%) but persisted with the addition of nonvascular deaths (relative risk reduction 24.1%, p = 0.023). Recurrence of stroke was more common in the placebo than in the ticlopidine group (p = 0.008), but the distribution of severity among these strokes was similar, as was the type of stroke suffered. An intention-to-treat analysis showed a 23.3% (1.0–40.5%; p = 0.02) relative risk reduction in stroke, MI or vascular death, confirming the benefit of ticlopidine.

Comment

This study shows that ticlopidine is of potential benefit in reducing the incidence of subsequent stroke, MI or vascular death in patients surviving a moderate or severe thromboembolic stroke. The primary analysis of efficacy was based on patients suffering stroke, MI and vascular death but excluding nonvascular deaths, and any events that occurred more than 28 days after the study drug was permanently discontinued, in order to increase clinical relevance and to make the assessment of efficacy more sensitive and accurate. The procedures for deciding about such exclusions were submitted for publication before the treatment code was broken [18]. Furthermore, no bias resulted from excluding ineligible patients or events after patients discontinued their study drugs. Confidence in the efficacy of ticlopidine is further strengthened by the consistency of benefit in different centers, for the two types of qualifying stroke (atherothrombotic or lacunar infarcts), for both men and women, and when based on an intention-to-treat as well as on an efficacy analysis.

Unwanted Effects in TASS and CATS

Overall in TASS, 62% of patients experienced some untoward reaction during the trial. Diarrhea was noted in 20% of patients on ticlopidine and in 10% of those on aspirin. Although 9% of the patients screened for TASS could not be randomized because of ASA intolerance or gastrointestinal bleeding in the previous 2 years, peptic ulceration, gastritis or bleeding occurred in over 2% of patients on ticlopidine and 6% of patients on ASA, among whom 2 deaths occurred after hematemesis. Maculopapular or urticarial rashes developed in 12% of patients on ticlopidine and in

5% of those on aspirin; none was life-threatening. After discontinuation of the drug the rash always resolved.

Severe neutropenia (absolute neutrophil count < 450/mm^3) developed in 8 women and 5 men taking ticlopidine between 1 and 3 months after starting the drug but cell counts returned to normal within 3 weeks of stopping ingestion in all cases. Mild to moderate neutropenia (absolute neutrophil count 450–1,200/mm^3) occurred in 22 patients on ticlopidine and in 12 on aspirin.

Patients on ticlopidine in TASS showed an increase in total plasma cholesterol levels from month 1, stabilizing to a mean increase of 11% over the initial (usually elevated) level by month 4, while the increase in aspirin-treated patients was 2%. The ratio of HDL to total cholesterol was similar in each treatment group. No change in the number of MIs occurred in the ticlopidine group.

Other Studies of Ticlopidine in Cerebrovascular Disease

Eight small trials of ticlopidine versus aspirin in the primary or secondary prevention of stroke have also been conducted, most of them in Japan. Only three were double-blind and randomized and all lasted a year or less; the total number of patients entered was less than 800. Reviewing these, I conclude that the value of small trials is limited, but where useful comparisons could be made, ticlopidine was superior to aspirin, much as was shown in the TASS trial. One small, double-blind trial in Japan [19] compared the effects of ticlopidine 200 mg and aspirin 500 mg daily, over a 12-month study period in 334 patients who had had TIAs in the previous 3 months. Review of the results showed that subjects taking ticlopidine had fewer (34 vs. 52) cerebrovascular events than those taking aspirin, although only the difference in the cumulative incidence of events over 3 years, including an open label study period, attained statistical significance (p = 0.036).

The Ticlopidine Microangiopathy of Diabetes Study (TIMAD) [20] was a randomized, doubly-masked, placebo-controlled trial designed to assess the effect of ticlopidine in reducing the progression of nonproliferative diabetic retinopathy in 435 IDDM patients over 3 years.

The mean yearly increase in definite microaneurysms shown by fluorescein angiograms was lower (p = 0.03) in the ticlopidine group. The drug yielded a sevenfold reduction in the yearly microaneurysm progression score compared with placebo (p = 0.03). The greatest inhibition of platelet aggregation was associated with cessation or reversal of microaneurysm progression, indicating an effect of the drug not only at the arterial but also at the arteriolar level.

Uchiyama et al. [21] performed the first trial of ticlopidine for the secondary prevention of TIA, using a dose of ticlopidine of 200 mg/day, which suppresses platelet aggregation in the average Japanese. The incidence of ischemic events was reduced by ticlopidine and in a subsequent double-blind multicenter trial of ticlopidine versus aspirin in patients with TIAs [22] the reduction in the incidence of subsequent stroke and MI was again significantly greater in patients treated with 200 mg ticlopidine than in those treated with 500 mg aspirin at 12 and 36 months after entry.

Uchiyama et al. [4] also used combination therapy with aspirin + ticlopidine in a further trial in 72 patients. The combination produced a greater prolongation of bleeding time (and more hemorrhagic complications) than did either agent alone and was considered to be a potent antiplatelet strategy, although the clinical importance of the changes observed were not described.

Discussion

The dose of aspirin employed in TASS was mandated by its official endorsement by USA regulatory authorities for the treatment of TIAs, following the Canadian trial [3]; in the circumstances, no alternative dose could be contemplated even though a lower dose is nowadays more frequently employed with more theoretical than practical justification. However, although the rate of unwanted effects with aspirin is dose-related, such a relationship is imperfect, as shown by examination of the side effects reported with different dosages in British trials [6, 9]. Although there may be no difference between the protective effects of 1,200 and 300 mg/day against disabling or fatal strokes and nonvascular deaths, there was a nonsignificant increase in the rate of intracerebral hemorrhage with the higher dose, although the numbers were very small. It should be noted that aspirin produced some unwanted effects more frequently than did ticlopidine even in low dosage.

Using the placebo data from the ESPS [15], the benefit of ticlopidine relative to placebo for nonfatal stroke or death from any cause can be estimated. In ESPS there was a 33% risk reduction achieved by the combination of ASA + dipyrimadole in nonfatal stroke or death at the end of the second year of the study. The cumulative event rate in TASS was 14.6 events. Using the ESPS figure, the 2-year cumulative effect of placebo should be 14.6 / 1-0.33 = 21.8 events. Using the estimated placebo rate to extrapolate an overall risk reduction achieved by ticlopidine, since the 2-year rate for ticlopidine was 11.6 events, the overall risk reduction ascribable to that drug is 21.8–11.6 / 21.8 = 47% which represents a substantial improvement over the benefit conferred by aspirin ingestion.

At the initiation of CATS the only evidence that aspirin was of value in the prevention of recurrent stroke was that from the Swedish trialists who considered it to be so on the basis not of their own results (which were not statistically significant), but on the results of a small meta-analysis which they performed on all such trials to date. Since then, other meta-analysis [11, 23] have also indicated a beneficial role of aspirin, insofar as they included among the trials analyzed a minority in which antiplatelet drugs were used following completed stroke. However, these indirect estimates and assumptions are made on the basis of different types of cerebrovascular event. The direct comparison of ticlopidine and aspirin has yet to be performed in the determination of the most effective therapy for patients who have suffered a completed stroke.

In the case of patients who have suffered TIAs, RINDs or strokes with minor residua, the comparison has been done (TASS), and demonstrates that ticlopidine confers superior protection, a benefit lost only when all results are pooled in meta-analysis and the TASS study compared with the composite of itself and all other trials.

One must be realistic about the absolute degree of protection afforded by the ingestion of any antiplatelet agent in patients at high risk. From the CATS figures for primary end-points, there were 29 fewer events among the 532 patients on ticlopidine. This represents an overall risk reduction of 22 or 30% over 3 years using ITT or efficacy analyses respectively, but only an average of 1.8% / year in the number of subjects who were spared an end-point. For the secondary CATS end-point of fatal or nonfatal stroke, the number of events avoided was 1.3% / year on average.

That males and females benefit equally from antiplatelet therapy was indicated by the ESPS [15] and AICLA [8] trial results and by meta-analysis [11], but in Canadian [3], Italian [24], and UK trials, benefit was restricted to males. That women have fewer TIAs, fewer strokes after TIA and a lower mortality rate anyway may be relevant. The TASS and CATS results show that ticlopidine is effective in both sexes.

Conclusion

In patients with atheromatous (or diabetic) vasculopathy, ticlopidine can reduce the risk of further serious events such as strokes. In studies comparing it directly with aspirin, ticlopidine has afforded a significantly greater protective effect, although initial meta-analytic studies have not demonstrated this. The relationship of the enhanced protection conferred by ticlopidine to its broader mode of platelet inhibition is speculative. The frequency of unwanted effects of ticlopidine is greater than that in patients taking aspirin and the unwanted effects themselves are different, although the rate of life-threatening complications is the same as that of aspirin. The risk-benefit ratio (comparing the number of permanent vascular events suffered with the risk of severe neutropenia) is firmly in favor of the use of ticlopidine. Probably in all patients, but especially in women and in those who cannot take or have failed to respond to aspirin, ticlopidine appears to be a useful agent for the prevention of secondary irreversible vascular events in patients shown to be at high risk as a result of its different mechanisms of platelet inhibition, its effects on small vessels, or both.

Zusammenfassung

Ticlopidin bei der Schlaganfallprophylaxe

Mehr als 20 Jahre wurde die Entdeckung von Craven [Miss Valley Med J 1952;74:213–215] ignoriert, bis die Canadian Cooperative Study Group [N Engl J Med 1978;299:53–56] den Nachweis erbrachte, daß Aspirin (ASS) das Risiko von Schlaganfällen und transitorischen ischämischen Attacken (TIA) bei symptomatischen Patienten verringert. Seither sind eine Reihe anderer Thrombozytenaggregationshemmer getestet worden, darunter Ticlopidin, das sowohl die primäre als auch die sekundäre Plättchenaggregation in Reaktion auf ADP, PAF und Kollagen, nicht jedoch auf Arachidonsäure hemmt.

Primärprävention: Jüngere Untersuchungen [N Engl J Med 1988;318:262–264; Br Med J 1988;296:313–316] legen nahe, daß ASS bei der Primärprävention möglicherweise das Risiko von Hirnblutungen erhöht; ASS bietet jedoch einen Schutz gegen Myokardinfarkte. Die schwedische Ticlopidin-Studie [J Intern Med 1990;227:301–308] zeigte bei Patienten mit Claudicatio intermittens innerhalb von 5 bis 7 Jahren keine signifikante Verringerung von Myokardinfarkten, Hirninfarkten und TIA. Die Gesamtsterblichkeit war jedoch vorwiegend durch Verringerung kardialer Todesfälle signifikant um 29,1% geringer als in der mit Plazebo behandelten Gruppe.

Sekundärprophylaxe: Metaanalysen von mehreren ASS-Studien bei Patienten mit TIA, RIND oder Insulten mit geringem neurologischem Defizit [Br Med J 1988;296:320–332] zeigen eine Risikoreduktion für Hirninfarkte, Myokardinfarkte oder vaskuläre Todesfälle mit einer Odds-Reduktion von $22 \pm 5\%$. Dies bedeutet, daß 73–83% derartiger Erkrankungen nicht verhindert werden. In der *Ticlopidine-Aspirin Stroke Study (TASS)* [N Engl J Med 1989;321:501–507] wurde der präventive Effekt von 2×250 mg Ticlopidin / Tag oder 2×650 mg ASS / Tag bei Patienten mit TIA, Amaurosis fugax, RIND oder Minimalinsult während 5,8 Jahren untersucht. Von 3069 Patienten wurden 1529 (1518 nahmen die Medikation) in die Gruppe, die Ticlopidin erhielt, und 1540 (1527 nahmen das Medikament) in die mit ASS behandelte Gruppe randomisiert. Das Durchschnittsalter betrug 63 ± 9 Jahre, zwei Drittel der Patienten waren Männer. 70% der qualifizierenden ischämischen Insulte wurden dem Karotisgebiet und 25% dem vertebrobasilären Stromgebiet zugeordnet. 52% der mit Ticlopidin und 47% der mit ASS behandelten Patienten brachen die Medikation ab. Mittels ITT-Analyse ergab sich für Ticlopidin eine Schlaganfallreduktion von 21% (Bereich 1–36%) und eine Reduktion von Schlaganfällen oder vaskulären Todesfällen von rund 8% (24 bis + 12%) gegenüber ASS. Kumulative Ereignisraten nach 12, 24 und 36 Monaten zeigten, daß die Wirkung im 1. Jahr besonders hoch war. Hierfür lassen sich zwei Ursachen anführen: die bekanntermaßen im 1. Jahr besonders hohe Insultrate nach einem Ersterignis und die Tatsache, daß die Population mit Risiko für einen Schlaganfall im Laufe der Jahre kleiner wird. Bei der Wirksamkeitsanalyse ergab sich über die gesamte Beobachtungszeit, daß 164 Patienten in der mit Ticlopidin behandelten Gruppe und 220 Patienten in der mit ASS behandelten Gruppe verstorben waren oder einen Schlaganfall erlitten. Tödliche und nichttödliche Schlaganfälle ereigneten sich bei 111 mit Ticlopidin und bei 165 mit ASS behandelten Patienten. Ticlopidin war bei der Schlaganfallprävention effektiver als ASS bei Patienten mit Karotissymptomen ohne hochgradige Karotisstenosen, aber weniger effektiv bei Patienten mit Stenosen $\geq 70\%$.

Da bisher keine eindeutigen Belege dafür vorliegen, daß ASS eine Wiederholung von Hirninfarkten verhindern kann [Stroke 1987;18:325–334], wurde in der *kanadisch-amerikanischen Ticlopidin-Studie (CATS)* [Lancet 1989;i:1215–1220] Ticlopidin gegenüber Plazebo getestet. 1072 Patienten wurden randomisiert; davon mußten 19 wegen Protokollverletzung ausgeschlossen werden. Für nichttödliche Schlaganfälle, nichttödliche Myokardinfarkte und vaskuläre Todesfälle ergaben sich in der mit Plazebo behandelten Gruppe 118 Ereignisse in 773 Patientenjahren (15,3% / Jahr); 74 Ereignisse in 683 Patientenjahren (10,5% / Jahr) wurden unter Ticlopidinbehandlung registriert. Ticlopidin bewirkte somit eine Risikoreduktion von insgesamt 30,2% (Bereich 7,5–48,3%). Die Reduktion betrug für Männer 28,1% und für Frauen 32,4%. Todesfälle aufgrund von anderen als vaskulären Ursachen und von Patienten, die länger als 28 Tage ihre Medikation nicht genommen hatten, wurden von der Analyse ausgeschlossen. Die Vorteile von Ticlopidin bleiben jedoch auch bei einer Intention-to-Treat-Analyse und bei Einschluß nichtvaskulärer Todesfälle bestehen.

Weniger umfangreiche Ticlopidin-Studien [z. B. Sang Thromb Vaisseaux 1990; 2:19–22] ergaben ähnliche Ergebnisse wie TASS. In einer plazebokontrollierten, randomisierten und doppelblinden Untersuchung [Arch Ophthalmol 1990;108:1577–1583] konnte nachgewiesen werden, daß Ticlopidin die Progression der nichtproliferativen diabetischen Retinopathie reduziert. Eine Verringerung oder sogar Umkehr der Progression war mit Plättchenaggregationshemmung assoziiert.

Unerwünschte Wirkungen – TASS und CATS: Insgesamt gaben 62% der Patienten Nebenwirkungen an. Durchfälle wurden bei 20% der Patienten unter Ticlopidin- und bei 10% der Patienten unter ASS-Behandlung beobachtet. Obwohl > 9% aller Patienten wegen ASS-Intoleranz oder gastrointestinalen Blutungen in den letzten 2 Jahren in TASS nicht randomisiert werden konnten, erlitten 2% der mit Ticlopidin und 6% der mit ASS behandelten Patienten peptische Ulzera, Gastritiden oder Blutungen, darunter 2 tödliche. Nach Absetzen der Medikation reversible makulopapulöse oder urtikarielle Effloreszenzen entwickelten 12% der mit Ticlopidin und 5% der mit ASS behandelten Patienten. Eine schwere Neutropenie (Anzahl neutrophiler Granulozyten < 450/mm^3) wurde nach 1–3 Monaten bei 8 Frauen und bei 5 Männern in der mit Ticlopidin behandelten Gruppe gefunden. Diese klang innerhalb von 3 Wochen nach Absetzen des Präparates ab. Leichte Neutropenien fanden sich bei 22 mit Ticlopidin und bei 12 mit ASS behandelten Patienten. Unter Ticlopidin kam es nach 4 Monaten zu einem mittleren Anstieg der Cholesterinkonzentration im Serum von 11%; unter ASS zu einem Anstieg von 2%. Myokardinfarkte waren in der mit Ticlopidin behandelten Gruppe nicht häufiger.

References

1   Craven LL: Prevention of coronary and cerebral thrombosis. Miss Valley Med J 1952;74:213–215.

2   Craven LL: Experiences with aspirin (acetylsalicylic acid) in the nonspecific prophylaxis of coronary thrombosis. Miss Valley Med J 1956;78:38–44.

3   Canadian Co-operative Study Group: A randomized trial of aspirin and sulfinpyrazone in threatened stroke. N. Engl J Med 1978;299:53–56.

4   Uchiyama S, Sone R, Nagayama T, et al: Combination therapy with low-dose aspirin and ticlopidine in cerebral Ischemia. Stroke 1989;20:1643–1647.

5   PHS Research Group. Preliminary Report: Findings from the aspirin component of the ongoing Physicians Health Study. N Engl J Med 1988;318:262–264.

6   Peto R, Gray R, Collins R, et al.: Randomised trial of prophylactic daily aspirin in British male doctors. Br Med J 1988;296:313–316.

7   Janzon L, Bergqvist D, Boberg J, et al: Prevention of myocardial infarction and stroke in patients with intermittent claudication: Effects to ticlopidine. Results from STIMS, the Swedish Multicentre Study. J Intern Med 1990;227:301–308.

8   Bousser MG, Eschwege E, Haguenau M, et al.: AICLA controlled trial of aspirin and dipyridamole in the secondary prevention of athero-thrombotic cerebral ischemia. Stroke 1983;14:5–14.

9   UK-TIA Study Group. United Kingdom Transient Ischemic Attack (UK-TIA) Trial: Interim results. Br Med J 1988;296:316–319.

10 The ESPS Group. The European Stroke Prevention Study (ESPS): Principal end-points: Lancet 1987;ii:1351–1354.

11 Antiplatelet Trialists Collaboration: Secondary prevention of vascular disease by prolonged antiplatelet treatment. Br Med J 1988;296:320–331.

12 Hass WK, Easton JD, Adams HP Jr, et al.: A randomized trial comparing ticlopidine hydrochloride with aspirin for the prevention of stroke in high-risk patients. N Engl J Med 1989;321:501–507.

13 Grotta JC, Norris JW, Kamm B, et al: Prevention of stroke with ticlopidine: Who benefits most? Neurology 1992;42:111–115.

14 Gent M, Blakely JA, Hachinski V, et al: A secondary prevention randomized trial of suloctidil in patients with a recent history of thromboembolic stroke. Stroke 1985;16:416–424.

15 ESPS Group. European Stroke Prevention Study. Stroke 1990;21:1122–1130.

16 Helmers C: High-dose acetylsalicylic acid after cerebral infarction. Stroke 1987;18:325–334.

17 Gent M, Blakely JA, Easton JD, et al: The Canadian-American Ticlopidine Study (CATS) in Thromboembolic Stroke. Lancet 1989;i:1215–1220.

18 Gent M, .Blakely JA, Easton JD, et al: The Canadian-American Ticlopidine Study in Thrombotic Stroke. Design, organization and baseline results. Stroke 1988;19:1203–1210.

19 Tohgi H: The Japanese ticlopidine study in transient ischemic attacks. Sang Thromb Vaisseaux 1990;2:19–22.

20 TIMAD Study Group: Ticlopidine treatment reduces the progression of nonproliferative diabetic retinopathy. Arch Ophthalmol 1990;108:1577–1583.

21 Uchiyama S, Osawa M, Maruyama M: Ticlopidine therapy in TIA and RIND (in Japanese). Gendai No Shinyro 1980;22:1325–1330.

22 Murakami G, Toyokura Y, Omae T, et al: Effects of aspirin and ticlopidine on transient ischemic attack (in Japanese). Sindan To Chiryo 1986;74:2255–2274.

23 Sze PC, Reitman D, Pincus MM, et al: Antiplatelet agents in the secondary prevention of stroke: Meta-analysis of the randomized clinical trials. Stroke 1988;19:436–442.

24 Candelise L, Landi G, Perone P, et al: A randomized trial of aspirin and sulfinpyrazone in patients with TIA. Stroke 1982;13:175–179.

Prof. W. E. M. Pryse-Phillips
Department of Neurology
Memorial University of Newfoundland
St. John's, NF A1B 3V6 (Canada)

Dorndorf W, Marx P (eds): Stroke Prevention.
Basel, Karger, 1994, pp 103–112

Ultrasound in Recognition, Epidemiology and Prevention of Atherosclerosis

A Preliminary Communication

G. Rudofsky

Angiologische Klinik, Universitätsklinikum, Essen, FRG

For nearly 15 years it has been possible to investigate structures and movements of organs with ultrasound imaging techniques. It of course permits the examination of vessels susceptible to ultrasound and therefore it also allows the early recognition of atherosclerosis.

At present, four different methods exist. With real-time scan the vessel walls and contents can be represented with high resolution [1, 3, 6, 12, 15, 22].

The two-dimensional technique, which is unsatisfactory for certain purposes, is now to be complemented by the three-dimensional method. Even complicated organic forms such as advanced plaques with their complex structure or tumors may be represented in their space relations [18].

The combination with pulsed Doppler ultrasound imaging allows additional assessment of blood flow. With modern electronic transducers it has become possible for the first time to make a really simultaneous assessment of the morphological real-time picture and the blood flow of individual parts of vessels, visualized on the ultrasound screen [20, 21]. This cannot be achieved with the mechanical working transducers, because the manual switch from Doppler to ultrasonic scanner jeopardizes the flow analysis since minor changes of the positioning of the transducer head may considerably deflect the pulsed Doppler from the desired site of examination [3, 8, 9, 15, 17.]

In angiodynography the whole picture is examined simultaneously with a Doppler flow analysis and the blood flow directions of all vessels perfused are represented on the screen. This technique still reduces the resolution of the picture, but probably also facilitates the demonstration of smaller vessels, e. g. in areas of the calf or acral sections, which to date cannot be represented by the other techniques due to overshadows of the scattered echo.

With real-time sonography it has become possible for the first time to examine vessel walls. Large-scatter devices may represent vessel changes of less than 1 mm of size. Thus, for example, atherosclerotic plaques of 1 µl volume may be measured. This method allows us to recognize early preclinical atherosclerosis in a noninvasive manner and to control its progression. An inpatient group of 600 patients without arteriosclerosis-caused diagnosis underwent routine sonographic examination of their carotid arteries, and a correlation was established between the incidence of plaques and the risk factors for atherosclerosis. Early manifestations such as signs of alterations and stenosing processes in the vessels appeared 20 respectively 10 years earlier in patients with multiple risk factors [16].

In another epidemiologic investigation in the frame of the Monica Project of the WHO, the time spent for ultrasound tests in prospective screenings of the carotid, femoral and popliteal arteries was measured (1,452 participants). All vessels could be investigated in about 15 min in the mean. Ultrasonic investigation might be a useful and reasonable instrument in early recognition of atherosclerosis. With increasing age a higher incidence of atherosclerotic lesions was found, in men about one decade earlier than in women [2]. Besides age there was a clear-cut correlation between carotid plaque formation and HDL fraction of total cholesterol, cigarette smoking, history of myocardial and cerebral infarction or diabetes mellitus. Weaker correlations could be shown for total cholesterol and hypertension. In women, significant correlations between cholesterol, hypertension and HDL could be found [5]. Atherosclerotic lesions in the femoral artery showed a correlation to total cholesterol. The atherosclerotic alterations in the popliteal artery proved no connections to the well-known risk factors.

Since 1981, we have been investigating if with real-time scanning it is possible to diagnose and control hemodynamically asymptomatic lesions of the vessel walls at an early stage [14]. Tests on the measurements of plaques, their reproducibility, as well as on experimental plaques in animals with clear-cut volumes, encouraged us to perform studies in asymptomatic probands with known risk factors [1, 3]. Especially in hypertensive patients, atherosclerosis is first localized near vascular bifurcations, where probably nutritional supply of the endothelial layers is impaired by high pressures laying on the vessel walls or recirculating turbulent blood flow with low diffusion gradients for nutritional needs.

A clearly different form is seen in patients with familiar hypercholesterinemia [19]. There a concentric cholesterol deposition ascending from the aortic arch to the carotid bifurcation can be seen.

Long-distance runners, who started practicing at advanced age, show an extended atherosclerosis of the superficial femoral arteries, supposing that volume overload in a not adapted vessel during long periods of exercise may also lead to a typical different form of atherosclerosis [11].

Early atherosclerosis shows poor echogenic subintimal vessel wall infiltrations. The wall thickening as described by some authors as initial finding could not be reproduced by others [1]. In the further course these infiltrations develop homogenous or heterogenous echoes, depending on their composition, but the surface to the vessel lumen seems to be still smooth. With sensitive devices the plaque composition can be differentiated in cholesterol, fibrin, coagulated blood or scar tissue [1]. Subendothelial bleeding shows the lowest to lacking echo density. In older infiltrations there might be condensation of the plaques with increasing echo density and shrinkage of the lesion and new infiltrations in close neighborhood. Calcium deposits in older plaques might be characterized by extinction of ultrasound behind them. The longer these infiltrates exist, the more heterogenous they will appear. In regions with extreme wall movement, as near the bifurcations or Hunter's channel, plaques might be sheared off and thrombi can form on their now rough surface. This can lead to embolism, stenosis and occlusion or in case of thrombus organization to a clinical silent wall lesion.

So different stages of the atherosclerotic plaque formation can be diagnosed with ultrasound and it is obvious that the possible influence of anti-atherosclerotic drugs depends on the mode of action of the drug and the individual possible stage of atherosclerosis and its underlying risk factors.

The early plaque has a geometrically definable form of a halfly ellipsoid disc and it therefore offers the possibility of long-term studies, because it can be easily measured and volume determined. This encouraged us in 1982 to start investigations in otherwise healthy patients with two or more risk factors for atherosclerosis in their history. At the initial control at least one nonexulcerative plaque must have been present in the examined vessel areas. Symptoms suggesting circulatory disorders of the heart, brain or extremities are criteria for exclusion.

The patients were recruited from an epidemiologic study on the incidence of vascular diseases in workers of the metal industry (total participants: 2,597) and a similar study in government clerks of the State of North Rhine-Westphalia and the community of Essen (4,087 participants up to now).

In several studies with identical design, to date 210 probands have been observed from 15 months to 4 years. They were examined with real-time scan at 3-month intervals, and the plaque volume was measured. The aim of the investigation was to study the development of atherosclerotic plaques. The following vascular regions were examined: the carotid artery in the extracranial course, the iliac, femoral and popliteal arteries on both sides, and the abdominal aorta.

In these studies two investigators repeated the measurements twice at 3-day intervals of 12 different plaques to confirm the reproducibility of the measured values. The 3-day intervals were chosen to limit the probability of spontaneous variations due to processes of transformation. The mean coefficient of variation was 14% in the first examination and 16% in the second examination; therefore, a satisfying reproducibility even of smaller plaques may be suggested. Also individual cross-comparison of plaque growth shows a similar development with respect to growth and regression. This means that the preconditions for long-term observations of atherosclerotic lesions were met with sufficient accuracy.

Typical patterns of distribution will be presented with the results obtained in a trial on the effect of a serotonin antagonist [14]. In the initial examination (n = 88) at the right carotid artery a total of 56 and at the left a total of 55 affected areas were found. Solitary changes were seen on the right in 32 cases and on the left in 28 cases. Multiple plaques were observed 24 times on the right and 27 times on the left. In the abdominal aorta a total of 12 alterations was observed, 3 of them were single and 9 multiple. In the iliac vessels plaques were diagnosed initially in 26 cases on the right and in 22 cases on the left (29 single, 37 multiple). In the femoral artery most changes showed on the right (29 single, 37 multiple) and 60 on the left (32 single, 28 multiple). In 16 cases changes at the popliteal artery were present: 16 single and 3 multiple changes on the right, and 14 single and 2 multiple on the left side.

This means that both sides are affected to the same extent as to plaque localization. The femoral and carotid arteries are the most affected vessels, the iliac artery coming after. The carotid or femoral artery always presented changes, while in the other examined vessels no isolated changes or new singular formations were seen during the observation period; these two vessels are the key arteries to diagnose atherosclerosis of the peripheral vascular system. For this reason, these vessels should always be examined together for recognition of early atherosclerosis, since isolated affection at one of them may occur.

The controls were carried out a 3-month intervals, and triple documentation was made as in the beginning. Each patient had his/her record on a separate videotape so that all examinations are documented in chronological order, and the ultrasonic device can be adjusted each time as in earlier examinations. Furthermore, the maximum length, width and height of all plaques were measured (in millimeters with two perpendicular planes for subsequent volume determination). The underlying hypothesis is that early atherosclerotic lesions have a semiellipsoidal shape, so the formula for semiellipsoid calculation was applied. In addition, the investigator documented in sketches the essential characteristics of the ultrasound picture, such as distances between vessel bifurcations, neighboring bony structures, and consistency of plaques. Exulceration of plaques or transition to stenosis to more than 40% were criteria for exclusion. In order to avoid further influences on the condition, the therapy was continued by the general practitioner.

When comparing the plaque growth in the two main localizations in long-term studies, there is less growth in the carotid than in the femoral artery, where the volume was found to have more than doubled within 20 months. In the follow-up period, in some probands the bigger plaques had a faster growth rate, regression and progression being almost synchronous when comparing both sides. Complete repair was seen in small plaques only. With this method it has become possible to control directly prevention effects in early atherosclerosis without clinical manifestation [7, 14].

Results

The following substances were applied: (a) placebo; (b) acetylsalicylic acid (ASA) at a dosage of 1.0 and 1.5 g/day; (c) ASA combined with dipyridamole (3×1 g/day), (d) naftidrofuryl 900 mg/day; (e) 'essential' phospholipids (EPL substance) for lipid reduction 2.7 g/day; (f) in a pilot study anipamil, a calcium channel blocker and 300 mg ASA/day.

In contrast to placebo, 1.5 g/day ASA increased the growth of plaques, possibly due to the antiphlogistic effect at this dose which inhibits natural repair processes at the plaques [4, 19]. At a lower dose of 1 g/day there was no difference as compared to placebo. In contrast to placebo, the combination of ASA and dipyridamole reduced the plaque growth; the difference, however, was not statistically significant which may be related to the small number of patients and/or shortness of observation period. Naftidrofuryl was able to produce a lasting delay of growth, probably due to the inhibiting action of serotonin receptors (H_2) [10]. Even 4 years afterwards, further reduction of growth was observed [14, 15].

In patients with disorders of the lipid metabolism, who in addition to diet required lipid-lowering treatment, a clear statistically significant reduction of growth was seen after 9–12 months of treatment with 'essential' phospholipids. This tendency to plaque reduction was seen also during the subsequent observation period (up to 18 months).

In contrast to the other test groups, under EPL treatment reduced growth and even decreasing volumes in particular of larger plaques (around 50 µl) were found. This appears to be surprising, but clear-cut considerations are necessary for the assessment of the overall result. Whereas in the other studies drug-requiring disorders of the lipid metabolism had been criteria for exclusion, these were the important criteria for inclusion in the phospholipid-treated group. It may be presumed that the plaques in this study were rich in cholesterol, susceptible to shrink in volume as a consequence of the lipid-lowering action of the test drug. Of course, the lipid content is less in small plaques, which explains the less marked effects. The statistically significant reduction in plasma cholesterol also supports this effect, especially since it occurs at an early moment and since an influence is possible just because of the favorable condition of reduced concentrations.

The increased plaque growth due to the 'classical' high-dose ASA of 1.5 g/day as compared to placebo has various explanations. With this excessive dose intramural hemorrhage into the plaques might have happened. However, the ultrasound test of our patients showed in no case signs of plaque bleedings [1]. Furthermore, the main criteria for entry into the study were not stenosing and not exulcerating alterations of the vessel walls. It may be presumed that at that stage thrombocyte aggregation is of minor importance for the progression of atherosclerosis; examinations of recent years, on the other hand, have shown that effective inhibition of aggregation in vivo is probably achieved at doses of 100–300 mg. At a daily dose of 1,500 mg the antiphlogistic effect of ASA is supposed to commence, which impairs physiological processes of limitation and absorption (i. e.

sterile inflammations) at the atherosclerotic plaque. This hypothesis is supported by the fact that at a dose of 1,000 mg/day no difference compared to placebo was found any more. At a dose of 900 mg/day combined with dipyridamole a growth reduction of the plaques, although not significant, was observed over a mean period of 18 months. A longer duration of the study might have yielded clearer results in this patient group.

According to recent investigations, local serotonin release and action on the arterial wall is of decisive importance in the formation of atherosclerosis [10]. It is a well-established fact that serotonin plays a role in the disruption of the cellular endothelium in the vascular intima; thus the vessel wall is damaged, which is supposed to be necessary for the formation of atherosclerosis. This process explains why serotonin inhibition by specific drugs, attacking principally at the H_2 receptors, may effectively delay the progression of atherosclerosis, as our investigations on naftidrofuryl suggest [14]. It is known that cholesterol deposition is an essential characteristic of atherosclerotic lesions. This deposition may be the consequence of scars at the vessel wall, but in the case of disorders of the lipid metabolism, cholesterol deposition may be excessive, or it may represent a special type of atherosclerosis in which cholesterol deposition is central.

In a first double-blind pilot study with a calcium channel blocker (anipamil) and aspirin in a dosage of 300 mg/day, there was a more pronounced regression (60 vs. 44%) and a slower progression (38 vs. 47%) under anipamil during an observation period up to 9 months in early atherosclerosis.

Zusammenfassung

Diagnose und Verlauf präklinischer Arteriosklerose und ihre Beeinflußbarkeit durch Medikamente

Die Analyse des Gefäßsystems mit darstellenden Ultraschalltechniken erlaubt Einblicke in die Frühstadien von Gefäßwanderkrankungen. Mit geeigneter Technik lassen sich atherosklerotische Plaques von 1 µl Volumen nachweisen. An 600 Krankenhauspatienten, die einer Routineuntersuchung der Karotiden unterzogen wurden, konnte nachgewiesen werden, daß Wandalterationen und Stenosierungen bei Patienten mit einzelnen oder multiplen Risikofaktoren 10 bzw. 20 Jahre früher nachweisbar werden [A. Schömig und W. Gekeler, Dissertation, Ulm, 1986].

Im Rahmen des Monika-Projektes konnte gezeigt werden, daß die Inzidenz der Atherosklerose mit dem Alter zunimmt, und zwar bei Männern etwa eine Dekade früher als bei Frauen. Dabei bestand eine starke Korrelation zwischen Karotisplaque-Formation und HDL-Fraktion, Zigarettenrauchen, Vorgeschichte mit Myokard- oder Hirninfarkt und Diabetes mellitus. Schwächere Korrelationen fanden sich für Gesamtcholesterin und Hypertonie. Bei Frauen fanden sich signifikante Korrelationen mit Cholesterin, Hypertonie und HDL-Fraktion.

Während atherosklerotische Läsionen der A. femoralis mit dem Gesamtcholesterin korrelierten, fanden sich für Veränderungen an der Poplitealarterie keine Verbindungen. Frühe Gefäßläsionen haben Risikofaktor-abhängiges Aussehen. Vor allem beim Hypertonus findet man Läsionen in Bifurkationen, wo die Nährstoffversorgung durch hohen Druck oder turbulente Strömung gestört ist. Bei familiärer Hypercholesterinämie zeigen sich dagegen zirkuläre Cholesterindepositionen vom Aortenbogen bis zur Karotisbifurkation.

Bei Langstreckenläufern, die erst in höherem Alter mit dem Laufen begonnen hatten, fanden sich ausgedehnte atherosklerotische Veränderungen an den Aa. fem. superficiales, vermutlich bedingt durch Volumenüberlastung.

Frühe Wandveränderungen bestehen in kaum echogenen subintimalen Wandinfiltrationen, eine von einigen Autoren beschriebene Wandverdickung konnte von anderen nicht gefunden werden. Im weiteren Verlauf entwickeln sich, abhängig von ihrer Komposition, homogene oder heterogene Echos, aber die Gefäßwandoberfläche ist weiterhin glatt. Mit sensiblen Aufnehmern kann die Zusammensetzung der Plaques (Cholesterin, Fibrin, koaguliertes Blut oder Narbengewebe) untersucht werden. Subendotheliale Blutungen haben die niedrigste oder gar keine Schalldichte. Kalziumdepositionen zeigen den bekannten Schallschatten. In Regionen starker Gefäßwandbewegungen können Plaques aufbrechen, die Oberfläche wird dann rauh.

An bisher 210 Probanden mit frühen atherosklerotischen Veränderungen (Ausschlußkriterien: Hinweise auf kardiale, zerebrale oder periphere Gefäßsymptome, exulzerierte Plaques und Stenosen > 40%) wurden

  a) Plazebo
  b) 1–1,5 g ASS
  c) ASS mit Dipyridamol (3×900 mg/Tag)
  d) 900 mg Naftidrofuryl pro Tag
  e) 2,7 g «essentielle» Phospholipide
  f) 300 mg ASS gegen Anipamil

hinsichtlich ihrer Wirkung auf Plaquewachstum untersucht.

1,5 g ASS/Tag beschleunigte das Plaquewachstum wahrscheinlich durch seine antiinflammatorische Wirkung (Inhibition natürlicher Reparationsprozesse). Plaqueblutungen wurden bei dieser Dosis nicht gesehen. 1 g ASS/Tag war im Vergleich zu Plazebo ohne Einfluß. ASS plus Dipyridamol verringerte das Plaquewachstum, allerdings nicht statistisch signifikant.

Naftidrofuryl bewirkte eine lang anhaltende Verzögerung des Plaquewachstums, die sich auch nach 4 Jahren fortsetzte. Der Effekt beruht möglicherweise auf einer Inhibition des Serotoninrezeptors (S2).

«Essentielle» Phospholipide reduzierten das Plaquewachstum bei Patienten mit Fettstoffwechselstörungen signifikant. Unterschiede zu gegenteiligen Ergebnissen in anderen Studien liegen wahrscheinlich daran, daß frühe Stadien untersucht wurden, in denen eine Erniedrigung der Plasmalipidwerte noch effektiv sein kann.

In einer doppelblind durchgeführten Pilotstudie wurden 300 mg ASS mit dem Kalziumblocker Anipamil verglichen. Es zeigte sich eine deutlichere Regression von Plaques (60 versus 44%) und eine langsamere Progression (38 versus 47%) unter Anipamil in einer Nachbeobachtungszeit von bis zu 9 Monaten.

Fazit

Ultraschalluntersuchungen eignen sich für die Früherkennung atherosklerotischer Veränderungen. Sie erlauben frühzeitige Verlaufsbeobachtungen und die Überprüfung der Effektivität von Maßnahmen der Primär- und Sekundärprävention. Es ergeben sich Hinweise darauf, daß Serotonininhibitoren die Progression der Atherosklerose hemmen.

Bei Patienten mit Hypercholesterinämie und Cholesterinplaques scheint eine geeignete Diät in Verbindung mit «essentiellen» Phospholipiden eine Verringerung des Plaquevolumens zu bewirken.

References

1   Cranley JJ Jr, Karkov WS, Baldridge ED: Atlas of duplex scanning: Carotid arteries. Philadelphia, Saunders, 1989.

2   DeMont-Hahn A: Ambulante Screeninguntersuchung der A. carotis, A. femoralis und A. poplitea mit der Real-Time-Sonographie an einem repräsentativen Bevölkerungsquerschnitt; Diss Ulm 1989.

3   Ehringer H, Bockelmann U, Konecny R, Koppensteiner L, Marosi E, Minar R: Schöfl Verschlusskrankheit der extracraniellen A. carotis: 'Spontanverlauf' und frühe Phase nach Thrombendarteriektomie im bildgebenden Ultraschall. VASA 1987;suppl 20:71–76.

4   Flower RJ, Moncada S, Vane JR: Analgesic-antipyretics and anti-inflammatory agents; in Gilman AG, Goodman LS, Rall ThW, Murad F (eds): The Pharmacological Basis of Therapeutics. New York, Macmillan, 1985.

5   Gostomzyk JG, Heller W-D, Stieber J, Rudofsky G, Hahn, Keil U: Gefässwandveränderungen und kardiovaskuläre Risikofaktoren – Ergebnisse einer B-Bild-Sonographieuntersuchung. Abstractband 25 Jahrestagung der DGSMP, 1989.

6   Hennerici M, Reifschneider G, Trochel V: Ultrasonic imaging of the carotid artery. A post-mortem study of 100 specimens. International Symposium on New Ultrasonic Methods in Cerebrovascular Disease, Freiburg 1982.

7   Hennerici M, Steinke W: Morphologie und biochemische Parameter zur Regression von Karotisläsionen. VASA 1987; suppl 20:77-84.

8   Imperato AM, Riles TS, Mintzer R: The importance of hemorrhage in the relationship between gross morphologic characteristics and cerebral symptoms in 376 carotid plaques. Ann Surg 1983;197:195–203.

9   Imperato AM: Carotid plaque pathology; in Boccalon H (ed): Angiologie. Paris, Libbey Eurotext, 1988.

10 Kessler CH, Hipp M, Voosen P, Mödder G, Petrovici J-N: Doppelisotopen-Szintigraphie der Halsgefässe bei Schlaganfallpatienten. Köln, 1987.

11 Rescher A, Nielen C, Egle M, Strube J, Ranft J, Rudofsky G: Arteriosklerotische Wandveränderungen als Ausdruck lokal einwirkender Dauerbelastung – Beobachtungen an den A. femorales bei Marathonläufern. VASA 1991;suppl 33:250.

12 Rudofsky G: Kompaktwissen Angiologie. Erlangen, Perimed, 1988.

13 Rudofsky G, Meyer P, Müller-Heyden E: Quantification of alterations of the vessel wall by real-time scan in vitro and in vivo. XIII World Congress of the International Union of Angiology, Rochester 1983.

14 Rudofsky G, Meyer P, Hirche H, Altenhoff B, Lohmann A: Erkennung und Verlaufskontrolle von frühen arteriosklerotischen Gefässläsionen. VASA 1987; suppl 20:165–169.

15 Rudofsky G: Duplexsonographie; in Driessmann A (ed): Aktuelle Diagnostik und Therapie in der Angiologie. Stuttgart, Thieme, 1988.

16 Schömig A, Gekeler W: Real-Time-Sonographie – eine rationelle Diagnostik zur Früherkennung arteriosklerotisch gefährdeter Patienten; Diss, Ulm, 1986

17 Sohn Ch, Rudofsky G: Die dreidimensionale Ultraschalldiagnostik – ein neues Verfahren für die klinische Routine? Ultraschall Klin Prax 1989;4:219–224.

18 Spengel F, Keller Ch: Atheromatöse Carotisveränderungen bei familiärer Hypercholesterinämie vor und nach Therapie. VASA 1991;suppl 33:55.

19 Strandness DE Jr: Exploration of cervicoencephalic circulation: Current state and future strategic trends; in Boccalon H (ed): Angiologie. Paris, Libbey Eurotext, 1988.

20 Van Damme H, Creemers E, Martin D, Demoulin JC, Limet R: Pathologic aspects of carotid plaques: surgical and clinical significance; in Boccalon H (ed): Angiologie. Paris, Libbey Eurotext, 1988.

21 Wheeler HB, Anderson FA: Can noninvasive tests be used as the basis for treatment of deep vein thrombosis? In Bernstein EF (ed): Noninvasive Diagnostic Techniques in Vascular Disease. St Louis, Mosby, 1985.

22 Zichner R, Weihrauch ThR: Zur optimalen Dosierung von Acetylsalicylsäure. Med Klin 1989;84:43–51.

Prof. Dr. G. Rudofsky
Direktor der Klinik für Angiologie
Universitätsklinikum Essen
Hufelandstraße 55
D-45122 Essen (FRG)

Dorndorf W, Marx P (eds): Stroke Prevention.
Basel, Karger, 1994, pp 113–121

Drug Inhibition of Atherogenesis: New Approaches

E. Betz

Institute of Physiology (I), Tübingen, FRG

Numerous strokes or transitory ischemic attacks are caused by occlusions or by progressing stenoses of the carotid arteries and their branches supplying the brain. The majority of carotid stenoses is based on atherosclerotic intimal proliferates in these arteries. Therapeutic measures are presently and mainly aimed at the prevention of destructions in brain tissue regions supplied by the stenosed arteries. Prevention of progression of atheromatous changes in the walls of the extracerebral arteries supplying the brain is usually restricted on recommendations obtained from data on the basis of epidemiological studies combined with experimental results obtained from hyperlipidemic rabbits.

Reopening of occluded or stenosed arteries or bypass operations are more frequently used in peripherial or coronary arteries than in arteries supplying the brain. There are several reasons for the somewhat not precisely aimed therapies to treat or inhibit genesis and progression of atherosclerotic plaques in brain-supplying arteries. One reason is the impossibility to continuously observe the development of carotid arteriosclerosis on its cellular basis in patients and to experimentally produce arteriosclerosis in man. Another reason lies in the danger for the brain tissue when one tries to reopen stenosed brain-supplying arteries with angioplastic techniques as they are frequently used in other parts of the artery tree.

Therefore, approaches for promising therapeutic and preventive measures have to be tried in in vivo or in vitro experiments. Arteriosclerosis is a multifactorial disease. The flowchart (fig. 1) gives an overview on the main factors participating in the development of lipid-containing athero-

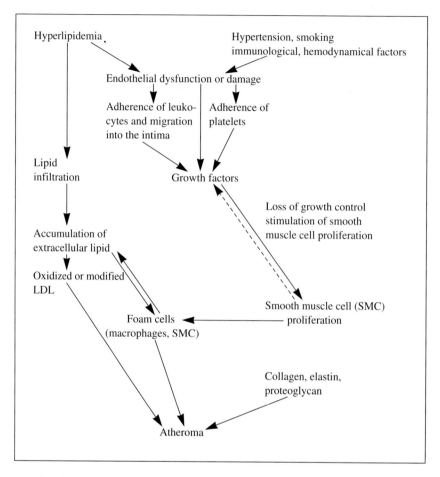

Fig. 1. Network of factors involved in the development of atheromas or fibromuscular proliferates. If no hyperlipidemia (left side of the diagram) exists, the proliferation is a fibromuscular intimal thickening.

mas or lipid-free intimal thickenings called fibromuscular proliferates. This diagram describes atherogenesis. However, it does not specifically regard the conditions for stenoses in brain-supplying arteries. In experiments in which the induction of hypercholesterinemia is induced by feeding the animals a diet with high cholesterol [1, 2] it could be seen that the first atheromas grew in the aorta and the coronary arteries. Later on, lipid depositions did not appear in the carotid arteries and its branches sometimes. Another method for the rapid production of an atheroma or a fibro-muscular proliferate in a carotid artery uses repetitive weak transmural electrical stimuli. In rabbits, 5 mm long and 0.2 mm wide graphite-coated gold electrodes are attached to the adventitia of a carotid artery in such a way that the stimulating current traverses the artery wall. From the electrodes, leads are conducted subcutaneously to a socket fixed in the skull and from there the electrodes can be connected to a stimulator with long leads so that stimulations are possible in the unrestrained animal. When the carotid artery of a rabbit is stimulated daily in the morning 30 min and again 15 min in the afternoon for 4 weeks, a subendothelial proliferate develops always at the anode side. With this technique the endothelial lining is not destroyed.

Most of the cells in the proliferate stain with antibodies against smooth muscle α-actin and against smooth muscle myosin. If the animal received during the 4 weeks' lasting experiment 0.5% cholesterol in its chow, the proliferate contained stainable lipid.

The stimulation technique enables to study all cellular components which are listed in the chart diagram (fig. 1) and to investigate the temporal development of an atheroma or an intimal fibromuscular proliferate in a carotid artery. When after the production of the stenosing carotid proliferate the stenosis is dilated with a balloon catheter or is removed by laser angioplasty, the development of a secondary stenosis can be easily studied. With this technique it is also possible to measure the effect of antiatherogenetic drugs as well as antiproliferative drugs. For this purpose we have standardized the stimulation procedure and used stimuli of 0.1 mA, 10 Hz, 15 ms/imp. every day 30 min in the morning and 15 min in the evening for 28 days. The cells arrange in layers so that the maximal number of cell layers in the subendothelial space can be taken as a measure of the thickness of the proliferate when the 6–8 mm long proliferate is sectioned in series.

In normal carotid arteries of rabbits the subendothelial space is void of cells so that all cells that appear within the intima must have migrated into the subendothelial space either from the blood or from the media. Kling [3] has analyzed the cellular composition of the proliferates during the development of the intimal thickenings and found that within the first days, granulocytes and mononuclear cells, mostly monocytes, appear in the subendothelial space within the irritated region. The granulocytes disappear after a few days and the relative and absolute number of monocytes decreases also and reaches at the end of the experiment approximately

Table 1. Effect of various substances on the proliferation of SMC in the intima of rabbit carotid arteries which were electrically stimulated daily with DC impulses of 0.1 mA, 10 Hz, 15 ms/imp. 30 min in the morning and 15 min in the evening during 28 days[1]

Substance	Dosis/day (mmol/kg b.w.)	Percent change of proliferation (growth) in comparison with untreated controls	Percent change of serum cholesterol in treated animals (comparison with untreated controls)	Percent change of serum triglycerides in treated animals (comparison with untreated controls)
Etofibrate	0.55 (po)	– 25 (NS)	– 15 (NS)	+ 80 (NS)
SP 54	0.003 (sc)	– 55 (S)	– 25 (NS)	+ 280 (NS)
Flunarizine	0.63 (po)	– 68 (S)	– 35 (NS)	– 30 (NS)
Verapamil	0.46 (po + sc)	– 48 (S)	– 5 (NS)	+ 50 (NS)
Nimodipine	0.24 (po)	± 0	+ 2 (NS)	– 4 (NS)

[1] The rabbits received during the 28 days 0.5% cholesterol in their food. As can be seen, there is no clear correlation between the changes of serum cholesterol and serum triglyceride levels and drug-induced reduction of the proliferation. po = Oral application; sc = subcutaneous application; S = significant; NS = not significant.

4–5% in rabbits fed a normal diet, whereas in cholesterol-fed animals the percentage of mononuclear cells can remain up to 25% of the total cell population. On the second day after onset of the stimulation a few smooth muscle cells (SMC) have already migrated through the pores of the elastic internal lamina into the subendothelial space where they undergo mitotic divisions. If a rabbit receives 3 days prior to the implantation of the electrodes 0.5% cholesterol in its food, the intima on the second day after beginning the experiment contains already macrophages with lipid-filled vacuoles. In contrast, the intimal cells of rabbits that received normal food do not contain lipid-filled vacuoles.

The stimulation technique has been widely used to study the actions of various antiatherogenetic drugs and it was found that very different substances are capable of inhibiting the formation of intimal proliferates. In table 1 it can be seen that there exists no direct relation between the effect of an antiatherogenetic drug on the development of the proliferate and on serum cholesterol or serum triglycerides of the rabbits. A dose-response curve of the calcium antagonist flunarizine shows a dose-dependent inhibition of the formation of a proliferate. However, a total stop of the proliferation could not be obtained with reasonable concentrations. This was seen with all the substances depicted in table 1.

Table 2. Effect of drugs which have been used for the inhibition of intimal proliferation in vitro experiments (see table 1) on the proliferation of vascular SMC and fibroblasts in mass cultures of cells: the SMC were obtained from arteries, the fibroblasts from sub-cutaneous tissue

Substance	Concen-tration mol/l	% inhibition of SMC prolifera-tion after 4 days of culture controls = no inhibition (= 0%)	% inhibition of fibroblast pro-liferation after 4 days of culture controls = no inhibition (= 0%)
Etofibrate	$8 \cdot 10^{-5}$	95	98
SP 54	$1.2 \cdot 10^{-5}$	62	0
Flunarizine, h	10^{-5}	37	42
Verapamil, h	10^{-5}	17	10
Nimodipine	10^{-5}	98	120

From animal experiments, conclusions with regard to the use of these substances for prevention or therapy of human atherosclerosis can be drawn only with some reserve. With in vivo studies it cannot be decided whether a substance inhibits proliferation because the applied concentration is toxic for the dividing cells. It is also difficult to clearly see if the drug inhibits specifically only those cell species which form the intimal proliferate and not also other cells, the mitosis of which should not be hindered. Finally, one cannot always be sure that an experimental animal reacts in an identical way to a drug as a patient. We have, therefore, combined the in vivo experiments with measurements of drug actions on cultures of cells obtained from human or animal vessels. For obtaining cells, pieces from bypass veins or from arteries were freed from endothelium and adventitia and were cut into small explants. These were laid on the bottom of collagen-coated Petri dishes and covered with culture medium. The outgrowing cells were isolated and used for testing drug effects in their 4th or 5th passage. Endothelial cells were obtained from human veins or animal arteries by enzymatic disaggregation. For tests with drugs added to the culture medium they were also used in their fourth passage.

The calcium antagonist flunarizine does not only inhibit human SMC but also EC in a concentration-dependent manner. The proliferation of fibroblasts is also inhibited. The calcium antagonist nimodipine inhibits also SMC and fibroblasts in culture, although it had no inhibitory effect on

Table 3. Inhibition in the development of proliferations in ballooned carotid arteries of rats with sulfated polyanions of the heparin-type and dextran sulfate[1]

Substance	DNA	Inhibition	Animals
	g/5 mm artery	%	n
Controls	3.82 ± 0.32	0	4
Heparin, type II			
(Sigma)	2.11 ± 0.08	45	4
Low-molecular heparin			
(4,300 daltons)	2.30 ± 0.39	40	4
Dextran sulfate	1.67 ± 0.32	56	4

[1] In comparison with normal heparin (Sigma) the anti-Xa activity of low-molecular heparin is low, so that high concentrations are tolerated by the animals. All substances were injected subcutaneously twice daily in a dosage of 1.5 mg/kg b.w.

the intimal proliferation in vivo as is demonstrated in table 1. Table 2 shows that with only one exception all substances that were demonstrated in table 1 did not specifically inhibit SMC growth. The exception is a polyanion which has a molecular weight of about 9,000 daltons. The experience with this substance (SP 54) stimulated us to search for drugs which did not affect EC grwoth or even stimulate EC proliferation and simultaneously inhibit SMC growth. Heparin has this effect. However, the natural heparins as well as SP 54 had such a strong anti-Xa activity that it seemed too risky to use the dosage necessary for a sufficient SMC inhibition in patients. We found a low molecular weight heparin (LMWH), molecular weight 4,000 D, which dose dependently inhibited human and animal SMC and stimulated EC proliferation also in a dose-dependent manner in vitro. Table 3 shows the concentration-response curves in cultures of human EC and SMC. The anti-Xa activity [15] is considerably lower than of natural heparin, so that high concentrations of the drug were successfully used in the described in vivo experiments.

When we found these promising results we produced proliferates in rabbit carotid arteries in the above-described way and reopened the stenosed carotid artery with a balloon catheter. The catheter was inserted into the common carotid artery proximally from the intimal proliferate and the balloon was placed into the stenosed artery section. After dilating the stenosed section with the inflated balloon, the catheter was deflated and removed. The responses of carotid arteries in animals which received for 4 weeks' daily subcutaneous injections of 4 mg/kg LMWH were compared with responses of carotid arteries in nontreated animals. The heparin treatment was started at the day when the artery was balloon-dilated. In histological sections of carotid arteries 4 weeks after ballooning the stenosed artery, one can usually see the border of the proliferate induced by electrical stimuli and a secondary stenosis after additional balloon treatment. In the nontreated animals the balloon dilatation always caused a massive secondary stenosis. Daily injections of LMWH for 7 days after ballooning inhibited the secondary proliferative activity considerably. In no case did the balloon dilatation of LMWH-treated animals cause a stroke. This may be partially caused by the anticoagulatory action of the drug. Table 3 shows the differences in plaque development of LMWH-treated and nontreated animals. In conclusion, the experiments demonstrate that it has become possible to reopen stenosed carotid arteries of rabbits and to suppress an excessive restenosis by the use of a drug therapy after angioplasty.

Zusammenfassung

Medikamentöse Hemmung der Atherogenese: Neue Wege

Die Arteriosklerose ist eine multifaktorielle Erkrankung, deren Pathogenese in vivo und in vitro untersucht werden kann. Hoher Cholesteringehalt in der Nahrung führt bei einigen Tierspezies zu Atheromen, die sich zuerst in der Aorta und in den Koronarien entwickeln, während Atherome der Karotiden oder ihrer Äste nur inkonstant beobachtet werden.

Eine Methode zur Erzeugung fibromuskulärer Proliferate oder Atherome an der Karotis wendet repetitive transmurale elektrische Stimulation an. Dabei werden Kaninchen-Karotiden durch 5 mm lange und 0,2 mm breite graphitbeschichtete Goldelektroden, die an die Adventitia angelegt werden, so gereizt, daß der Stimulationsstrom (0,1 mA, 10 Hz, 15 ms) die Arterienwand durchdringt. Die Stimulationen erfolgen morgens während 30 min und nachmittags während 15 min über einen Zeitraum von 4 Wochen. Dadurch entwickelt sich an der Anodenseite immer eine subendotheliale Proliferation. Die meisten dieser Zellen lassen sich mit fluoreszierenden Antikörpern gegen glattmuskuläres α-Aktin und α-Myosin anfärben. Werden die Tiere zusätzlich mit 0,5% Cholesterin in der Nahrung gefüttert, enthalten die Proliferate auch anfärbbare Lipide. Nach neueren Untersuchungen [Kling; in Hoffmeister, Betz (Hrsg.): Wechselwirkungen zwischen Blut und Gefäßwand; Tübingen, Attempo-Verlag, 1989, pp 95–109] wandern in den ersten Tagen Granulozyten und mononukleäre Zellen, vorwiegend Monozyten, in den subendothelialen Raum der irritierten Region. Die Granulozyten verschwinden nach einigen Tagen, und auch die absolute Zahl der Monozyten verringert sich. Am Ende des Experiments machen Monozyten bei Kaninchen unter Normaldiät etwa

4–5% der Zellen aus. Bei Tieren mit cholesterinreicher Nahrung können Monozyten jedoch bis zu 20% der gesamten Zellpopulation ausmachen. Schon am 2. Tag nach Beginn der Stimulation sind einige glatte Muskelzellen durch Poren der Lamina elastica interna in den subendothelialen Raum gewandert, wo sie zahlreiche Mitosen zeigen. Bei Tieren, die schon 3 Tage vor Implantation der Elektroden 0,5% Cholesterin in der Nahrung erhielten, fanden sich Makrophagen mit lipidhaltigen Vakuolen. Die Stimulationstechnik ist benutzt worden, um den antiatherogenen Effekt von Medikamenten zu untersuchen. Für Etofibrat, SP 54, Flunarizin und Verapamil ließen sich konzentrationsabhängige Proliferationsverminderungen von zwischen 25 und 68% nachweisen, die keine direkte Korrelation mit dem lipidsenkenden Effekt dieser Medikamente aufwiesen. Eine völlige Unterdrückung war jedoch mit vertretbaren Dosen nicht erreichbar. Nimodipin wies bei Kaninchen keinen proliferationshemmenden Effekt auf, weil der First-pass-Effekt sehr stark ausgeprägt war.

Von Tierexperimenten können nur sehr beschränkt und vorsichtig Rückschlüsse auf die Verhältnisse beim Menschen gezogen werden. Vor allem ist es sehr schwierig zu differenzieren, ob der Antiproliferationseffekt nur die Zellen im Proliferat betrifft und nicht auch andere Zellen, wie z. B. Endothelzellen, Fibroblasten, Epithelzellen usw., deren Wachstum nicht behindert werden soll.

Aus diesem Grunde wurden zusätzlich Untersuchungen an Zellkulturen aus menschlichen Gefäßwänden durchgeführt. Dazu wurden Stücke von Venen oder Arterien, die bei Bypassoperationen gewonnen wurden, von Endothel und Adventitia befreit und in kollagenbeschichteten Petri-Schalen mit Kulturmedium bedeckt. Auswachsende Zellen wurden isoliert und der Medikamenteffekt während der 4. bis 5. Passage der kultivierten Zellen gemessen. Endothelzellen wurden von menschlichen Venen und Arterien oder Tierarterien durch enzymatische Disaggregation gewonnen. Zur Testung wurden die Medikamente dem Kulturmedium beigefügt und der Effekt während der 4. Passage bestimmt. Dabei zeigte sich, daß der Kalziumantagonist Flunarizin nicht nur die Proliferation von glatten Muskelzellen und Fibroblasten, sondern auch die von Endothelzellen dosisabhängig hemmt. Ähnlich verhielten sich Etofibrat, Verapamil und Nimodipin, obwohl letzteres in vivo bei Kaninchen keinen antiproliferativen Effekt gezeigt hatte. Das Polyanion SP 54 mit einem Molekulargewicht von 9000 Dalton hemmte die Proliferation von glatten Muskelzellen spezifisch, ohne Fibroblasten oder Endothelzellen ebenfalls zu hemmen.

Die Ergebnisse mit dieser Substanz stimulierten die Suche nach Substanzen, die spezifisch das Wachstum glatter Muskelzellen hemmen, das Wachstum von Endothelzellen aber nicht behindern, sondern sogar stimulieren. Derartige Effekte lassen sich für Heparine nachweisen. Leider haben die natürlichen Heparine in der zur Proliferationshemmung erforderlichen Konzentration eine so starke anti-Xa-Aktivität, daß ihre klinische Anwendung zu risikoreich scheint. Ein niedermolekulares Heparin mit einem Molekulargewicht von 4000 zeigte eine dosisabhängige Hemmung der Proliferation glatter Muskelzellen bei gleichzeitiger Stimulation des Enthelzellwachstums. Da seine anti-Xa-Aktivität deutlich geringer war, konnte eine In-vivo-Anwendung in hohen Dosen durchgeführt werden. Hierzu wurden bei Kaninchen in der beschriebenen Weise Proliferate an der Karotis erzeugt und dann die entstandene Stenose durch Ballondilatation erweitert. Der Effekt von 4 mg/kg niedermolekularem Heparin, täglich subkutan während 4 Wochen appliziert, wurde mit unbehandelten Kontrollen verglichen. Dabei zeigte sich eine deutliche Verringerung der Proliferate und somit eine Hemmung der bei den Kontrollen erheblichen Restenosierung. Bei den mit Heparin behandelten Tieren kam es bei keiner Ballondilatation zu einem Hirninfarkt, was teilweise an der mäßig ausgeprägten gerinnungshemmenden Wirkung liegen könnte.

References

1   Anitschkow N, Chalatow S: Über experimentelle Cholesterinsteatose und ihre Bedeutung für die Entstehung einiger pathologischer Prozesse. Z Allg Pathol Pathol Anat 1913;24:1–14.
2   Wissler RW: Neueste Studien über die Pathogenese und Rückbildung der Atherosklerose. Therapiewoche 1982;32:3735–3745.
3   Kling D: Interaktion von Leukozyten und Arterienwand in der Frühphase experimenteller Arteriosklerose; in Hoffmeister, Betz (eds): Wechselwirkungen zwischen Blut und Gefässwand. Tübingen, Attempto-Verlag, 1989, pp 95–109.

Prof. Dr. E. Betz
Direktor des Physiologischen Instituts
Eberhard-Karls-Universität Tübingen
Gmelinstraße 5
D-72076 Tübingen (FRG)

Surgical and Interventional Prevention

Dorndorf W, Marx P (eds): Stroke Prevention.
Basel, Karger, 1994, pp 122–130

Surgical Complications of Carotid Endarterectomy

J. van Gijn

University Department of Neurology, Utrecht, The Netherlands

The two randomized trials of carotid endarterectomy in symptomatic patients that have been completed in the past year have dramatically changed the position of this operation, though at this moment perhaps more in scientific standing than in clinical practice. Both studies showed that in patients with severe carotid stenosis (linear diameter reduced by 70–99%) the risk of disabling or fatal stroke decreases spectacularly after carotid endarterectomy, from 11 to 6% after 3 years in the European Carotid Surgery Trial (ECST) [1], and from 13 to 4% after 2 years in the North American Symptomatic Carotid Endarterectomy Trial [2]. Perioperative strokes are included in these percentages, and the immediate risks of the operation had been 'won back' (for the operated patients as a group) after as short a period as 1 year (fig. 1). In contrast, for patients with a degree of stenosis under 30%, who were randomized only in the European study, the risk of subsequent stroke was so low that even after 3 years the losses from perioperative stroke outweighed any benefit. For patients with intermediate degrees of stenosis, both trials continue the follow-up of randomized patients and the entry of new patients.

This clear-cut positive result from the two trials has two important implications. First, carotid endarterectomy is indicated in patients with a transient ischemic attack or a nondisabling ischemic stroke in whom the angiogram shows a stenosis between 70 and 99%, *provided the expertise of the surgical team in question is comparable to that of the teams who took part in the trials.* Second, now that the operation is here to stay, efforts should be doubled to make it more safe. This is the subject of my contribution. Perioperative strokes are the most dreaded complications and I shall

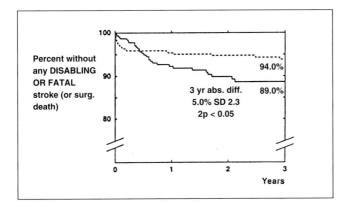

Fig. 1. Life-table analysis of patients with severe carotid stenosis (reduction of linear diameter by 70–99% on the prerandomization angiogram), randomly allocated to 'surgery' (28/455; broken line) or 'no surgery' (33/323; solid line). For the group of operated patients, the losses from perioperative stroke or death are compensated not at the point in time where the two lines cross, which is after slightly less than 6 months, but only after the two lines have diverged over an area equal in size to that contained between them before the point of crossing. Even so, the net balance of surgery becomes positive within 1 year, at least for the average surgeon who participated in the trial. [Data and fig. from 1, with permission from Lancet.]

therefore concentrate on these. I shall add a brief section about injuries of peripheral nerves associated with carotid endarterectomy; such nerve injuries are not disabling but may yet substantially affect the quality of life.

Rates of Perioperative Stroke

In the European centers which took part in the ECST, the total rate of perioperative death or stroke (defined as focal deficits producing symptoms for more than 1 week) was 7.5% on average; half of this proportion (3.7%) applied to deaths or disabling strokes (with disability 6 months later) [1]. In general, there is a great variation in the rate of perioperative stroke or death, between 2 and 25% [3, 6]; the range must be even wider if centers are included which do not publish their results. In addition, the crude rate of perioperative stroke depends not only on *how* the operation is done but also *in whom* it is done. The operation is much safer in asymptomatic patients, with 'inactive arteries', but the diagnosis of a transient ischemic attack is notoriously difficult [7]. Some surgeons include a mythical category of 'carotid stenosis with nonhemispheric symptoms', which in my view should be read as 'asymptomatic carotid stenosis with a history of overbreathing or some other unrecognized and unrelated disorder'. In addition, the rate of perioperative stroke depends on the *definition of stroke*. For instance, 'major stroke' is defined by some as anything lasting longer than 1 week [8], by others as disability persisting up to 3 months [2].

In the past, several measures have been proposed to decrease the risk of stroke after carotid endarterectomy: intraoperative monitoring (by a variety of methods), maintenance of an adequate blood pressure, and insertion of a shunt for the period that the internal carotid artery is clamped (routinely, or on the basis of measurement of the stump pressure after application of the proximal clamp). Although these measures have been adopted by many surgeons, controlled clinical trials in support of this are ostensibly lacking, and some skeptical surgeons regard all monitoring and shunting as superfluous. But before randomized trials are mounted in this field, it is appropriate to consider the *pathogenesis* of perioperative stroke in more detail than is usually the case in surgical reports.

Pathogenesis of Perioperative Stroke

First of all, what are the relative proportions of ischemic and hemorrhagic strokes after carotid endarterectomy? Intracerebral hemorrhages after carotid endarterectomy have been associated with high-grade stenosis, reduced perfusion pressure and uncontrolled hypertension [9], but hemorrhages account for only a small minority of perioperative strokes. One series reported intracerebral hemorrhage after 0.5–1% of all operations [10]. Hemorrhages were even more rare among the first 90 perioperative strokes in the ECST [unpublished and preliminary results; I shall repeatedly refer to this series]; of the 54 patients investigated by early CT scanning, a hemorrhage was found in only 1, and that in the opposite hemisphere.

The most important distinction within the group of perioperative strokes is therefore not that between hemorrhages and infarcts, but between infarcts resulting from a low-flow state, caused by clamping or thrombosis, and thromboembolism, resulting from manipulation of the diseased artery or from thrombosis of the repaired artery. This distinction can be made on the basis of several criteria (table 1).

Table 1. Factors that can help in distinguishing between low-flow state and thromboembolism in the analysis of perioperative infarction

Interval between coming round from the anesthetic and stroke
Intraoperative monitoring
Predisposing factors
Pattern of infarction on CT
Re-exploration of the artery
Autopsy after fatal perioperative strokes

If a neurologic deficit is caused by hemodynamic factors, it should be apparent when the patient comes round from the anesthetic, but of course not all immediately postoperative strokes can be attributed to this cause. In contrast, if ischemic stroke occurs after an *interval* of hours, days or even weeks (the limit of the postoperative period is arbitrarily set at 30 days), thromboembolism is the most likely explanation. Such an interval after the operation was found in 11 of 34 perioperative strokes in a retrospective series from the Netherlands [11], and in 43 of the 90 ECST patients with perioperative stroke.

EEG *monitoring* during surgery often but not invariably detects intraoperative stroke; particularly subcortical infarcts may not be reflected by focal changes in the EEG. If the development of asymmetry coincides with clamping the problem is probably but not invariably hemodynamic [11]; the alternative explanation is that pressure from the clamp releases one or more emboli. The study of intraoperative embolization has received new impetus from the technique of *transcranial Doppler ultrasonography*. In about half of all operations this new tool shows evidence of embolization in the middle cerebral artery, often repetitive and sometimes massive [12, 13]. The release of emboli is associated with manipulation or penetration of the artery, such as insertion of a needle (for measurement of the stump pressure or for injections), insertion of a shunt, closure or release of a clamp, or application of adhesive plaster to the wound. Particularly release of the distal clamp may give rise to a continuing stream of emboli, which probably represents the washing away of debris from the arterial wall. Such massive embolization may be followed by ischemic deficits [13]. On some occasions the surgeon is able to stop the stream of emboli by adapting his technique, guided by the auditory feedback from the transcranial Doppler machine [13]. An additional advantage of transcranial Doppler monitoring is that this technique can also detect hemodynamic phenomena, in the form of substantial flow reductions in the middle cerebral artery, before EEG changes occur – or sometimes without these.

Predictive factors for perioperative stroke have been preliminarily analyzed for the ECST. Baseline factors associated with perioperative stroke were female sex (smaller size of arteries?), a systolic blood pressure over 180 at randomization, peripheral vascular disease, and a high level of cholesterol; the last three factors probably reflect the severity of atherosclerosis. The same applies to the predictive factors 'TIA of the brain' (and not of the eye) and 'severe or moderate stenosis' (as opposed to mild stenosis), which directly represent the severity of carotid disease. Operation-related factors associated with perioperative stroke were a duration over 2 h, shunt insertion (both probably indicate severe involvement of the artery rather than faulty technique), perioperative hypo- or hypertension, and, interestingly, advoidance of anticoagulant drugs.

The most important evidence in the distinction between hemodynamic and thromboembolic infarction is *the pattern of infarction on the CT scan*. Previous studies have shown that hemodynamically induced infarcts often occur in the shape of borderzone infarcts, either between the cortical territories of the major cerebral arteries, or between the cortical and the perforating branches of the middle cerebral artery [14, 15]. Only if the diminution of cerebral blood flow is generalized and long-lasting the ischemic changes on the CT scan are bilateral or even diffuse. In contrast, infarcts within the territory of a cortical artery (complete or partial) are considered of thromboembolic origin. Surprisingly, very few studies have addressed this issue, presumably because neurologists have not been closely involved with the management of postoperative stroke. For the ECST series not all scans have yet been collected, as far as these have been made. In the retrospective series from the Netherlands, only 7 of the 34 perioperative strokes were hemodynamically induced, as judged from the CT scan [11].

Exploration of the operated artery in case of perioperative stroke is of course not systematically performed. In 10 of the 90 cases from the ECST a Fogarty catheter was introduced or the wound was reopened, and in only 4 of these local thrombus was found. Autopsy, in 4 patients from the ECST series, showed complete occlusion by thrombus, mostly up to the middle cerebral artery, but obviously fatal cases are not representative for perioperative stroke in general.

Damage to Cranial or Peripheral Nerves

Cranial nerve palsies after carotid endarterectomy are not rare; in one prospective series the rate was 15% [16]. The hypoglossal nerve is most commonly affected, permanently in one third of the patients. This paralysis gives rise to difficulties in speaking and swallowing. Damage to the recurrent laryngeal nerve, resulting in vocal cord paralysis with hoarseness, is the next most common cranial nerve injury. Recovery is the rule [16], but there are exceptions [17]. The lower division of the facial nerve is more rarely involved, with a deficit in movement of the lower face. These three branches of the twelfth, tenth and seventh nerve all traverse the carotid artery at some level, and it has been maintained that most damage can be avoided by dissection close to the arterial wall [16]. On the other hand, these nerves can also be caught in the retractor [17].

Cutaneous nerve damage usually involves the greater auricular nerve, transverse cervical nerve, or both. This was found in more than half the patients in one series [17], and is difficult to avoid. Some of these patients remain troubled by numbness or by pins and needles.

Conclusions

To conclude: (1) Hemorrhage is a rare cause of perioperative stroke; (2) at least three quarters of perioperative infarcts are thromboembolic in origin, if account is taken of circumstantial evidence from (a) the interval between operation and stroke; (b) intraoperative monitoring, particularly transcranial Doppler ultrasonography; (c) the pattern of infarction on CT scanning; (3) a good operative technique is necessary to avoid not only strokes, but also damage to cranial nerves, and finally (4) published complication rates are not generalizable to surgical teams in general. Within institutions, surgical performance should be carefully audited, and compared with the results achieved in the European and North American trials [18].

Zusammenfassung

Chirurgische Komplikationen der Karotisendarteriektomie

Die beiden randomisierten Untersuchungen über die Karotisendarteriektomie (CEA) bei symptomatischen Patienten haben bei hochgradigen Stenosen (70–99% lineare Durchmessereinengung) eine deutliche Verminderung behindernder oder tödlicher Schlaganfälle von 11 auf 6% nach 3 Jahren im European Carotid Surgery Trial [Lancet 1991;337:1235–1243] und von 13 auf 4% im North American Symptomatic Carotid Endarterectomy Trial [N Engl J Med 1991;325:445–453] nachgewiesen. Patienten mit hochgradigen symptomatischen Stenosen sollten aber nur unter der Voraussetzung operiert werden, daß die Erfahrung des Operationsteams mit derjenigen der an den Untersuchungen beteiligten Zentren vergleichbar ist. Darüber hinaus sollten die Anstrengungen zur Verminderung der Operationskomplikationen verdoppelt werden.

Perioperative Schlaganfälle. In der europäischen Untersuchung war die Rate aller perioperativen Todesfälle und Schlaganfälle (definiert als fokales Defizit mit Symptomen von mindestens einer Woche Dauer) 7,5%; die Hälfte davon entfiel auf tödliche oder auch noch nach 6 Monaten behindernde Schlaganfälle. Generell werden in der Literatur Komplikationsraten zwischen 2 und 25% angegeben. Ob diese zentralnervalen Komplikationen durch geeignete perioperative Überwachung, Aufrechterhaltung eines adäquaten Blutdruckes oder Shunt-Insertion verringert werden können, ist eine offene Frage.

Pathogenese operativer Schlaganfälle. Intrazerebrale Blutungen nach CEA sind mit 0,5–1% selten [Eur J Vasc Surg 1987;1:51–60]. Im European Trial fand sich unter den ersten 90 perioperativen Insulten nur eine Blutung, die noch dazu kontralateral lokalisiert war.

Ischämische perioperative Insulte können Resultat einer *Mangelperfusion* durch Abklemmung oder Thrombose sein oder auf *Thromboembolien* infolge der Manipulation an der Gefäßwand oder Thrombosen in der Reparaturphase zurückgeführt werden. Eine Differenzierung gelingt durch Beachtung folgender Kriterien: a) Intervall nach Beendigung von Operation und Narkose; b) Intraoperative Überwachung; c) Prädisponierende Faktoren; d) Infarktmuster im CCT; e) Reexploration der Arterie; f) Autopsie bei Verstorbenen.

Ein hämodynamisch verursachter Insult sollte sofort nach Beendigung der Operation bzw. Narkose evident sein. Ein derartiger zeitlicher Zusammenhang beweist jedoch nicht eine hämodynamische Genese. Insulte, die mit zeitlicher Latenz von Stunden, Tagen oder sogar Wochen eintreten, dürften eher auf thromboembolische Mechanismen zurückzuführen sein. Ein derartiges Intervall wurde in einer holländischen Serie [Stroke 1989;20:324–328] bei 11 von 34 perioperativen Schlaganfällen und in 43% der 90 perioperativen Insulte im ECST gefunden.

Die EEG-Überwachung kann oft, aber keinesfalls immer, intraoperative Schlaganfälle aufdecken. Koinzidieren fokale EEG-Veränderungen mit der Abklemmung, ist eine hämodynamische Genese wahrscheinlich. Alternativ kommt aber auch eine Embolisation thrombotischen oder atheromatösen Materials durch die Abklemmung in Frage. Eine vielversprechende Überwachungsmethode ist mit dem transkraniellen Doppler gegeben, der nicht nur Embolisationen während der Abklemmung und vor allem unmittelbar nach Lösung der distalen Klemme gut nachweisen kann, sondern auch hämodynamische Mangelsituationen vor EEG-Veränderungen aufdecken kann.

Prädiktive Faktoren für perioperative Insulte sind im ECST untersucht worden. Eine Assoziation fand sich mit weiblichem Geschlecht (geringere Arterienweite?), einem systolischen Blutdruck über 180 mm Hg bei Randomisierung, peripherer Verschlußkrankheit und hohem Cholesterinwert. Diese letzten drei Faktoren dürften die Schwere der Arteriosklerose reflektieren. Gleiches gilt für die prädiktiven Faktoren «schwere oder mittelgradige Stenose» (im Gegensatz zu «leichte Stenose») und TIA des Gehirns (nicht des Auges). Operationsbezogene Faktoren waren Dauer der Operation über 2 h, Shunt-Insertion, perioperative Hypo- oder Hypertension und Vermeidung von Antikoagulantien.

CCT-Muster sind für bestimmte Hirninfarktmuster indikativ. Grenzzoneninfarkte als typische Zeichen eines hämodynamisch verursachten Infarktes fanden sich in der niederländischen Serie in nur 7 von 34 perioperativen Infarkten. Daten für ECST liegen bisher nicht vor.

Nicht bei allen perioperativen Insultfällen erfolgte die Exploration operierter Arterien. Im ECST wurden nur 10 von 90 Arterien exploriert. Dabei fanden sich lokale Thromben nur bei 4. Zusätzlich liegen autoptische Untersuchungen von 4 Patienten vor; alle vier wiesen Thrombosen auf, die meist bis in die A. cerebri media reichten. Dies scheint aber nicht generell repräsentativ für perioperative Insulte zu sein.

Insgesamt läßt sich aus allen verfügbaren Zusatzdaten ableiten, daß zumindest drei Viertel aller perioperativen Schlaganfälle embolisch bedingt sind.

Neben den zentralnervalen perioperativen Schädigungen dürfen Läsionen peripherer Nerven nicht vergessen werden; diese finden sich in etwa 15% der Fälle [Stroke 1984;15:157–159]. Sie betreffen vor allem den N. hypoglossus, seltener den N. recurrens oder den unteren Fazialisast. Läsionen der Hautnerven (N. auricularis magnus, N. transversus colli) kommen in etwa 50% der Fälle vor und sind oft nicht zu vermeiden.

References

1   European Carotid Surgery Trialists' Collaborative Group: MRC European Carotid Surgery Trial: interim results for symptomatic patients with severe (70–99%) or with mild (0–29%) carotid stenosis. Lancet 1991;337:1235–1243.

2   North American Symptomatic Carotid Endarterectomy Trial Collaborators: Beneficial effect of carotid endarterectomy in symptomatic patients with high-grade carotid stenosis. N Engl J Med 1991;325:445–453.

3   Warlow C: Carotid endarterectomy: Does it work? Stroke 1984;15:1068–1076.

4   Dyken M, Pokras R: The performance of endarterectomy for disease of the extracranial arteries of the head. Stroke 1984;15:948–950.

5   Toronto Cerebrovascular Study Group: Risks of carotid endarterectomy. Stroke 1986;17:848–852.

6   Lusby RJ, Wylie EJ: Complications of carotid endarterectomy. Surg Clin North Am 1983;63:1293–1302.

7   Koudstaal PJ, van Gijn J, Staal A, Duivenvoorden HJ, Gerritsma JGM, Kraaijeveld CL: Diagnosis of transient ischemic attacks: Improvement of interobserver agreement by a checklist in ordinary language. Stroke 1986;17:723–728.

8   UK-TIA Study Group. United Kingdom Transient Ischemic Attack (UK-TIA) Aspirin Trial: Final results. J Neurol Neurosurg Psychiatry 1991;54:1044–1054.

9   Caplan LR, Skillman J, Ojemann R, et al: Intracerebral hemorrhage following carotid endarterectomy. Stroke 1978;9:457–460.

10 Schroeder T, Sillessen H, Boesen J, Laursen H, Soelberg Sorensen P: Intracerebral hemorrhage after carotid endarterectomy. Eur J Vasc Surg 1987;1:51–60.

11 Krul JMJ, van Gijn J, Ackerstaff RGA, Eikelboom BC, Theodorides T, Vermeulen FEE: site and pathogenesis of infarcts associated with carotid endarterectomy. Stroke 1989;20:324–328.

12 Spencer MP, Thomas GI, Nicholls SC, Sauvage LR: Detection of middle cerebral artery emboli during carotid endarterectomy using transcranial Doppler ultrasonography. Stroke 1990;21:415–423.

13 Jansen C, Vriens EM, Eikelboom BC, Vermeulen FEE, van Gijn J, Ackerstaff RGA: Carotid endarterectomy with transcranial Doppler and electroencephalographic monitoring: a prospective study in 130 operations. Stroke 1993;24:665–669.

14 Ringelstein EB, Zeumer H, Schneider R: Der Beitrag der zerebralen Computertomographie zur Differentialtypologie und Differentialtherapie des ischämischen Großhirninfarktes. Fortschr Neurol Psychiat 1985;53:315–336.

15 Torvik A: The pathogenesis of watershed infarcts in the brain. Stroke 1984;15:221–223.

16 Massey EW, Heyman A, Utley C, Haynes C, Fuchs J: Cranial nerve paralysis following carotid endarterectomy. Stroke 1984;15:157–159.

17 Dehn TCB, Taylor GW: Cranial and cervical nerve damage associated with carotid endarterectomy. Br J Surg 1983;70:365–368.

18 Barnett HJM: Stroke prevention by surgery for symptomatic disease in carotid territory. Neurol Clin 1992;10:281–292.

Prof. J. van Gijn, MD, FRCPE
Department of Neurology
University Hospital Utrecht
NL–3508 GA Utrecht (The Netherlands)

Dorndorf W, Marx P (eds): Stroke Prevention.
Basel, Karger, 1994, pp 131–143

Current State of Carotid Endarterectomy

O. Busse

Department of Neurology, Klinikum Minden, FRG

Introduction

After the first successful carotid reconstruction in 1954 [1], carotid endarterectomy (CEA) became enormously popular. In North America this procedure was one of the most commonly performed operations. The hopes and expectations of CEA are that removing an atherothrombotic embolic source to the brain and, in cases of severe stenosis, improving cerebral blood flow and reactivity, would reduce the risk of stroke. There have been many optimistic surgical reports without adequate controls but not conclusive proof of the efficacy of this procedure. The negative results of two randomized studies [2, 3] were totally ignored and the frequency of the operation raised from year to year. In the last 10 years the enthusiasm for CEA tempered because of the following reasons: The perioperative risk in an individual case is often unpredictable and dependent on the selection of patients. Therefore, the perioperative morbidity and mortality, as reported in the literature, varied between 2.5 and 20%. Before considering a CEA it is important to know that after the onset of ischemic warning symptoms the chance of dying from heart disease, principally myocardial infarctions, is greater than a fatal stroke. We must also know that the only representative study of Fields et al. [2] in 1970 was performed without medication of antiplatelet drugs, which are able to prevent stroke. The angiography, in our opinion still necessary before operation, is a small but a definite risk even in experienced centers. The risk of stroke and death should be no more than 1% [4, 5]. All these facts led to controversial discussions regarding the indication for CEA. Therefore, two randomized studies aimed at establishing clearer indications for CEA were performed in recent years.

Results of the European Carotid Surgical Trial (ECST) [6] and the North American Symptomatic Endarterectomy Trial (NASCET) [7]

In summer 1991 the first interim results of the two randomized multi-center CEA studies were published. The results were very similar in both studies. In summary the conclusion is that CEA for high-grade symptomatic carotid stenosis (70–99%) is highly effective in preventing subsequent ipsilateral strokes. Furthermore, the ECST provides no direct support for carotid surgery in patients with mild stenosis (0–29%).

The design of both studies was very similar, therefore the results are comparable. Eligible were patients with a carotid territory nondisabling ischemic stroke, transient ischemic attacks (TIA's) and retinal infarctions within the previous 6 months (ECST) and 120 days (NASCET) in association with probable significant ipsilateral stenosis of 0–99% (ECST) and 30–99% (NASCET). The measurement of carotid stenosis in both studies was different. In NASCET the ratio of the narrowest diameter of the diseased artery to the diameter of the artery beyond the bulb is measured, in ECST the ratio of diameter of carotid stenosis to the diameter of the bulb was measured. Therefore, an overestimation of the stenosis in ECST is probable. In ECST only patients were eligible if the neurologist and surgeon were absolutely uncertain whether to operate or not. On the other hand, if the doctors were certain in their approach, the patients were not eligible. It was our experience as one of the participating centers that we were rarely sure whether CEA would work or not and therefore most of the patients with symptomatic carotid artery stenosis were randomized.

There was no substantial difference in the exclusion criteria [6, 7]. In ECST between 1981 and 1991 a total of 2,200 patients were randomized in the ratio 60% surgical and 40% medical therapy. The median time between randomization and operation was 12 days, the mean duration of follow-up was 2.7 years.

In NASCET the randomization ratio was 1 : 1. The operation was performed in an average of 2 days after randomization, the mean follow-up duration was 1.5 years. In both ECST and NASCET all patients got the best available conservative therapy including antiplatelet, antihypertensive drugs, etc.

Table 1. Perioperative risk for death and stroke in ECST and NASCET: death and stroke rate in NASCET for the comparable 32-day period after randomization in the medically treated patients

Events	ECST (70–99%)		NASCET (70–99%)				ECST (0–29%)	
	surgical (n = 455)		surgical (n = 328)		medical (n = 331)		surgical (n = 219)	
	n	%	n	%	n	%	n	%
Death any cause	4	0.9	2	0.6	1	0.3	3	1.4
Death + all stroke	34	7.5	18	5.8	11	3.3	10	4.6
Death + major stroke	17	3.7	7	2.1	3	0.9	5	2.3

Results

Symptomatic Severe Stenosis (70–99%)

The perioperative risk within 30 days after operation for death and major stroke in patients with severe carotid stenosis was 3.7% (ECST) and 2.1% (NASCET). The complication rate regarding all stroke and death was 7.5 and 5.8% (table 1). In NASCET the rate of stroke in the comparable 32-day period – CEA was performed within a mean time of 2 days after randomization – was in patients with conservative therapy as expected much lower. The perioperative risk for death and all strokes was relatively high with 4.6% and for death and major stroke with 2.3% in the patients with a mild stenosis.

In ECST patients with severe (70–99%) stenosis showed after an apparently successful surgery about an 8-fold reduction in ipsilateral ischemic strokes (5/455 vs. 27/323). Including all perioperative complications and all major and fatal strokes and cerebral bleedings there is still a benefit to be gained from the operation (28/455 vs. 33/323). Figure 1a shows that the cross-over point with risk balance between surgical and medical therapy lies at 6 months. The main benefit may be in the first year because later on the curves run in a parallel course.

More impressive are the results in NASCET (table 2). The risk of any fatal or nonfatal ipsilateral stroke within 24 months after randomization

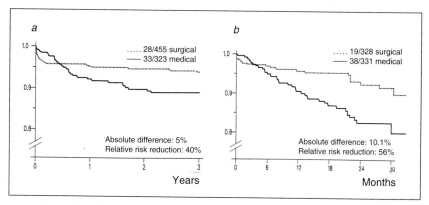

Fig. 1. Life-table analysis (survival curves) for all disabling or fatal strokes including surgical death of any cause in ECST *(a)* and NASCET *(b)*.

Table 2. NASCET: Number of events within 2 years of follow-up for six definitions

Events	Medical (n = 331)		Surgical (n = 328)		Absolute difference, %	Relative risk reduction, %
	n	%	n	%		
Any ipsilateral stroke	61	26.0	26	9.0	17.0	65
Any stroke	64	27.6	34	12.6	15.0	54
Any stroke or death	73	32.3	41	15.8	16.5	51
Major ipsilateral stroke	29	13.1	8	2.5	10.6	81
Any major stroke	29	13.1	10	3.7	9.4	72
Any major stroke or death	38	18.1	19	8.0	10.1	56

was 26% for the medical patients and only 9% for the surgical ones. Thus, for every 100 patients treated surgically, 17 were spared an ipsilateral stroke in the next 2 years. Therefore, 6 patients are the number needed to be treated to prevent one event within 24 months. Table 2 shows that CEA remains beneficial with respect to each of the five other definitions of outcome events. Figure 1b shows that the early disadvantage of the surgical patients, because of perioperative stroke and death, was rapidly overcome with the curves for the medical and surgical patients crossing already about 3 months after randomization.

There was a correlation between the risk reduction and degree of stenosis. The absolute risk reduction of all ipsilateral strokes was 26% in patients with 90–99% stenosis, 18% with 80 89% and 12% with stenosis of 70–79%.

In both studies the risk of ipsilateral stroke in the medical group was unexpectedly high – 16.8% in 3 years in ECST and 26% in 2 years in NASCET. But if the patient survives surgery without complications the stroke risk in the next few years is not completely abolished but very low.

Moderate Stenosis (30–69%)

The results in NASCET as in ECST are still unclear and therefore both studies are continuing.

Mild Stenosis (0–29%)

This group of patients was examined only in ECST. Neither for ipsilateral stroke nor for all disabling and fatal strokes was there any substantial or significant difference between surgically and medically treated patients. Important is the result, that there are almost no ipsilateral ischemic strokes to be prevented.

Clinical Approach for CEA Indication

The questions which arise include: Are these results generalizable? Is it mandatory to perform a CEA in all patients with a carotid territory TIA or minor stroke and severe stenosis of the carotid artery? What can really be concluded from the results of ECST and NASCET?

The relatively low perioperative risk is due to the participation of selected surgeons, who have a high level of experience in CEA. The surgical risk rate in both studies should be a guideline for surgeons. The recommendations of the Stroke Council, American Heart Association [8] permitted higher risk rates: For TIAs and ischemic stroke a combined morbidity and mortality rate of 5 and 7% was suggested. If the perioperative risk exceeds the rate of 2.1 and 3.7% for major stroke and death, the benefit of CEA will diminish. If the rate of major complications exceeds the guidelines of the Stroke Council, the benefit will vanish entirely.

Significance of Carotid Lesion

In our opinion it is by no means always justified to perform a CEA if a severe carotid stenosis is combined with transient ischemic symptoms or minor stroke in the corresponding carotid territory. The doctor who decides the indication must be sure that the carotid stenosis is significant, that means is responsible for the ischemic symptoms. Almost 20% of strokes are caused by emboli from the heart, and in older patients nonvalvular atrial fibrillation with thrombus formation in the left atrium is not rarely coexistent with a high-grade carotid stenosis. In these cases it can be very difficult to confirm the real pathogenesis of the ischemic event. Echocardiography and Holter monitoring are often helpful in differential diagnosis. Nearly one third of ischemic strokes are caused by lacunes due to hyalinosis in deep perforator arteries (small vessel disease, microangiopathy). Probably it makes no sense to perform a CEA in a patient with a widespread microangiopathy of the brain. On the other hand, Millikan and Futrell [9] stressed that a lacunar stroke can be caused by a small intra-arterial and cardiac embolus as well. In the ECST study a CCT was not mandatory, but in the NASCET study it was. It would be interesting to review the CCTs in respect to lacunes and to evaluate the results of these patients.

Activity of Carotid Lesion

Ischemic cerebral symptoms in patients with carotid stenosis are more often caused by arterial embolism than by hemodynamic changes. Therefore, it seemed wise to find criteria for active, emboligenic carotid lesions. The importance of ulceration or hematoma in carotid plaques is controversial [10, 11]. Sometimes the indium-111-platelet scintigram can be helpful in detecting active carotid plaques [12, 13]. Perhaps turbulences and retrograde flow in the Doppler flow color imaging are signs for active lesions with an unfavorable spontaneous course of the carotid atherosclerotic process [14]. In conclusion, we do not yet have strong criteria for active lesions' to predict the stroke risk.

Perioperative Cardiac Risk

The association between carotid and coronary artery diseases is well known and lies at approximately 50%. The leading course of death of patients with cerebral infarctions and TIAs is myocardial infarction rather than recurrent stroke. Cardiac complications of endarterectomy can be minimized by avoiding or delaying CEA in patients with a recent myocardial infarction or instable angina pectoris. All patients have to be evaluated for coronary artery disease very carefully before CEA. A standard ECG and Holter monitoring should be routinely performed. Other tests are an echocardiography for detecting ventricular dysfunction, stress ECG and thallium-myocardial scanning. A new method is the dipyridamol-thallium imaging for patients who are unable to undergo a maximal stress test [15, 16]. Dipyridamol, like strenuous exercise, causes marked coronary vessel dilatation and a general increase in coronary blood flow. Whether patients with no evidence of coronary disease and normal standard ECG and Holter monitoring should also have the stress tests before CEA is still controversial. In unstable angina pectoris, recent myocardial infarction and pathological stress tests, a coronary angiography is recommended.

In general it is not recommended to perform a simultaneous operation of symptomatic coronary and carotid atherosclerotic disease, because it is associated with higher morbidity and mortality [16]. The carotid surgery should be performed prior to coronary artery surgery. Exceptions are suggested for patients with active neurological symptoms and bilateral carotid lesions in conjunction with unstable coronary artery disease. Indeed, the neurological complications can be very high.

Timing of CEA

In ECST and NASCET the interval from onset of ischemic symptoms to the randomization was 6 months and 120 days. The efficacy of carotid surgery is unknown if the interval is longer. If the patient was asymptomatic after an ischemic event for 1 year or longer, it is justified to treat him medically.

What is the best time for operation after the ischemic event? In our experience a patient with TIA without signs of ischemic infarction in CCT or MRI can be operated on some days after the event. It is wise to delay carotid surgery for a few weeks after a recent stroke with infarction in imaging and if the patient is neurologically unstable. An ipsilateral intracerebral hemorrhage can occur due to postoperative hyperperfusion in a recently ischemic region.

Asymptomatic Carotid Stenosis

The prophylactic CEA of an asymptomatic carotid stenosis is a controversial issue. In the literature there is no agreement concerning stroke risk of these patients. Patients with moderate stenosis have an annual risk of 0.9–1.7% [17, 18]. If the stenosis exceeds 80% or is rapidly progressing, the annual stroke risk increases to about 5% [18]. It was suggested that stroke in asymptomatic carotid stenosis is mostly preceded by warning TIA but that is not true in all cases. Like symptomatic patients the risk for myocardial ischemia is much higher than for ischemic stroke [17, 18]. In an unrandomized study, Moneta et al. [19] showed that patients with high-grade asymptomatic carotid stenosis and CEA have a better outcome than nonoperated patients. The data in the literature about mortality and neurological morbidity are different; the complication rate should not exceed 3% as recommended by the Stroke Council of the American Heart Association [8].

Until now no randomized study about efficacy of CEA in asymptomatic patients existed. Now the results of the German Casanova study (*Carotid Artery Stenosis with Asymptomatic Narrowing: Operation versus Aspirin*) were published [20]. 410 patients with uni- and bilateral symptomatic carotid stenosis between 50 and 90% were randomized. There was no difference in the outcome in both groups. The perioperative mortality and major stroke rate was 3.2%, a value comparable with the perioperative risk in ECST and NASCET. These results suggest that even in experienced centers there is no indication for a prophylactic CEA in patients with asymptomatic carotid stenosis less than 90%. Three other studies for asymptomatic carotid stenosis [21–23] are in progress. Perhaps they will help to clarify this issue, although it is by no means certain that this will be the case.

If prophylactic CEA is not undertaken, a close follow-up with clinical and ultrasound evaluation is necessary. The patient and the physician have to be sensitive for warning ischemic symptoms and progression of the carotid stenosis. But there are some exceptions in which prophylactic CEA can be performed.

CEA can be justified in patients with clinically silent infarction, revealed by cerebral imaging and ipsilateral high-grade carotid stenosis. CEA can also be discussed in severe (more than 80%) or progressive stenosis if the cerebral vascular reactivity measured by transcranial Doppler CO_2 or intravenous Diamox test is impaired [24]. Therapy of bilateral asymptomatic carotid stenosis/occlusion remains to be defined. The measurement of cerebral vascular reactivity can facilitate the decision. But patients with multivessel disease have a more widespread atherosclerosis with coexistent coronary disease and therefore an increased perioperative risk. Young adults without coronary disease have a lower spontaneous and perioperative risk for myocardial ischemia and should be operated on.

A common practice at least in cardiovascular surgical departments is the prophylactic CEA in conjunction with major cardiovascular surgery. This is mostly undertaken in coronary artery bypass surgery (CAB). Significant extracranial carotid disease is present in 5–10% of patients with coronary artery disease [25]. The overall stroke incidence for cardiac surgery is low and appears to increase in patients with asymptomatic carotid stenosis, although exact data are missing. Performing CEA prior to or simultaneous with major vascular reconstruction (CAB, aortic surgery) is based on the premise that hemodynamic changes during surgery predispose to stroke in case of a carotid stenosis. But clear proof that prophylactic endarterectomy will decrease neurological morbidity is lacking. In many centers nowadays it is usual to perform CAB and CEA simultaneously [26]. At present there are insufficient data to support the policy of a simultaneous versus staged surgical approach. In general, CEA should be performed prior to cardiac surgery. The decision for CEA should be made on the same basis that is used in patients without known cardiac disease.

Conclusions

To conclude: (1) The ideal candidate is a patient with acceptable cardiac risk, who has had one or more carotid territory TIAs or minor stroke and a severe atherosclerotic lesion at the appropriate carotid bifurcation. (2) An absolute condition is the clinical significance of the carotid lesion for the ischemic cerebral symptoms. (3) Patients with acute ischemic stroke and disabling symptoms are not appropriate candidates for CEA. (4) Patients with mild stenosis should not be operated on. In ECST there is a trend against surgery. (5) In patients with moderate carotid stenosis the balance of surgical risk and medical therapy remains unclear. Both ECST and NASCET will continue. In unstable carotid disease CEA can be indicated. (6) Asymptomatic carotid stenosis generally is no indication for CEA. Close clinical and ultrasound follow-up is necessary. Possible exceptions are silent infarctions in imaging, high-grade and progressive stenosis, bilateral carotid stenosis, young adults without coronary disease and major cardiovascular surgery.

Zusammenfassung

Gegenwärtiger Stand der Karotisendarteriektomie

Symptomatische Karotisstenosen: Die hohe Frequenz der Karotisendarteriektomie (CEA) in einigen Ländern kontrastierte zu den negativen Resultaten früherer prospektiver Untersuchungen [JAMA 1970;211:1993–2003, J Neurol Sci 1984;64:45–53], zumal auch in späteren Jahren perioperative Komplikationsraten zwischen 2,5 und 20% zu verzeichnen waren. Wegen der Indikationsunsicherheit wurden zwei prospektive randomisierte Untersuchungen durchgeführt, deren Zwischenergebnisse jetzt vorliegen: der European Carotid Surgery Trial (ECST) [Lancet 1991;25:1235–1243] und der North American Symptomatic Endarterectomy Trial (NASCET) [N Engl J Med 1991;325:445–453]. In beide Studien wurden Patienten mit nicht behindernden oder passageren ischämischen Insulten und/oder retinalen Infarkten innerhalb der letzten 6 Monate (ECST) oder 120 Tage (NASCET) aufgenommen, wenn eine korrespondierende Karotisstenose von 0–99% (ECST) oder von 30–99% (NASCET) vorlag. Als Maß des Stenosegrades wurde im ECST das Verhältnis Durchmesser der Stenose zu Durchmesser des Bulbus caroticus, im NASCET das Verhältnis Durchmesser der Stenose zu Durchmesser der Carotis interna jenseits des Bulbus verwendet. Der ECST randomisierte von 1981 bis 1991 2200 Patienten zu operativer bzw. allein medikamentöser Therapie in einem Verhältnis von 60 zu 40%, NASCET randomisierte 662 Patienten (70–99% Lumeneinengung) in einem Verhältnis von 1 : 1. Die durchschnittliche Nachbeobachtungszeit beträgt beim ECST 2,7, beim NASCET 1,5 Jahre.

Symptomatische schwere Stenosen: Das perioperative Risiko (innerhalb von 30 Tagen nach Operation) ist in Tabelle 1 im Text dargestellt. Nach erfolgreich überstandener CEA ergab sich im ECST eine 8fache Reduktion von ipsilateralen Schlaganfällen gegenüber der nur medikamentös behandelten Gruppe (5/455 bzw. 27/323). Auch bei Berücksichtigung der perioperativen Komplikationsrate verbleibt der Vorteil für das Kollektiv der Operierten (28/455 bzw. 33/323). Abbildung 1 im Text zeigt, daß die durch perioperative Komplikationen bedingte anfängliche Risikoerhöhung in der Gruppe der Operierten schon nach 6 Monaten umschlägt: Der Kreuzungspunkt der Überlebenskurven frei von Schlaganfall der beiden Kollektive liegt bei etwa 6 Monaten. Der größte Vorteil für die Operation scheint im ersten Jahr zu liegen, da später die Kurven annähernd parallel verlaufen. Die Ergebnisse des NASCET (Tab. 2, siehe Text) zeigen ein noch positiveres Ergebnis: Bei 100 Operationen ergab sich eine Verringerung von 17 ipsilateralen Schlaganfällen in 2 Jahren. Der Kreuzungspunkt der Überlebenskurven frei von Schlaganfall liegt bei etwa 3 Monaten. Leider liegen für mittelgradige Stenosen (30–70%) z. Zt. noch keine klaren Ergebnisse vor, so daß beide Studien fortgesetzt werden. Bei niedriggradigen Stenosen (0–30%) ergab sich im ECST kein Vorteil für die Operation, d. h. das perioperative Risiko wurde im Langzeitverlauf nicht aufgeholt.

Für die Indikationsstellung zur CEA ergaben sich folgende Konsequenzen: Die chirurgische Komplikationsrate darf – auch wenn die Empfehlungen des Stroke Councils der American Heart Association [Circulation 1989;79:472–473] etwas höhere Komplikationsraten für vertretbar halten – nicht wesentlich höher sein als in den genannten Studien. Die Karotisstenose muß mit hinreichender Sicherheit Ursache der Symptome des Patienten sein. Dies ist zweifelhaft bei begleitenden embolisch wirksamen Herzerkrankungen (z. B. Vorhofflimmern, intrakavitären Thromben) oder prädominierender zerebraler Mikroangiopathie. Die

Bedeutung von Ulzerationen und subintimalen Blutungen als Indikatoren emboligener Aktivität ist nicht eindeutig bekannt. Kardiale Komplikationen im Rahmen einer CEA können durch Voruntersuchungen [EKG, 24-Stunden-EKG, Belastungs-EKG, Echokardiographie und Dipyridamol/-Thallium-Szintigraphie] vorhergesehen und wahrscheinlich verringert werden. Simultane Operationen an Koronarien und Karotis sind wegen der hohen Komplikationsrate nicht zu empfehlen. Nur bei symptomatischen Patienten mit hochgradigen ein- oder beidseitigen Karotisstenosen und instabiler Angina pectoris werden Ausnahmen diskutiert. Der Zeitpunkt der Operation nach einem ischämischen Ereignis sollte nicht jenseits von 6 Monaten oder 120 Tagen liegen. Bei transitorischer ischämischer Attacke ohne Infarktzeichen im kranialen Computertomogramm kann die CEA schon nach wenigen Tagen durchgeführt werden. Bei Hirninfarkten sollte die CEA erst nach wenigen Wochen erfolgen.

Asymptomatische Karotisstenosen: Die CEA bei asymptomatischen Stenosen ist umstritten. Bei mittelgradigen Karotisstenosen ist das spontane Hirninfarktrisiko mit 0,9–1,7%/Jahr sehr gering, bei Stenosen von ≥ 80% und bei progredienten Stenosen mit 5%/Jahr deutlich höher [Brain 1987;110:777–791, N Engl J Med 1986;315:860–865]. Die einzige bisher veröffentlichte prospektiv randomisierte Studie [Stroke 1991;22:1229–1235] zeigte bei einer perioperativen Komplikationsrate (Tod oder schwerer Schlaganfall) von 3,2% keinen Vorteil für die CEA bei Patienten mit Stenosen < 90% Lumeneinengung. Z. Zt. laufen drei prospektive Untersuchungen [Stroke 1989;20:844–849, Mayo Clin Proc 1989;64:897–904, Stroke 1986;17:534–539], von denen man eine Klärung der Operationsindikation erhoffen kann. Angesichts der Unsicherheit der Operationsindikation läßt sich eine CEA im asymptomatischen Stadium nur bei Stenosen ≥ 80% Lumeneinengung, progredienten Stenosen, Stenosen mit korrespondierendem stummem Hirninfarkt, bilateralen hochgradigen Stenosen und einseitigen Stenosen bei jungen Erwachsenen ohne Koronarerkrankung rechtfertigen. Die Indikation zu einer prophylaktischen CEA vor oder simultan mit einem koronaren Bypasseingriff ist umstritten. Etwa 5–10% dieser Patienten haben begleitende signifikante Karotisstenosen. Die Schlaganfallrate bei koronarer Bypasschirurgie ist generell gering, scheint aber bei Karotisstenoseträgern höher zu sein. Dennoch ist die Wirksamkeit einer prophylaktischen CEA in diesem Zusammenhang bisher nicht belegt.

References

1   Eastcott HHG, Pickering GW, Rob CG: Reconstruction of internal carotid artery in a patient with intermittent attacks of hemiplegia. Lancet 1954;ii:994–996.

2   Fields WS, Maslenikov V, Meyer JS, Hass WK, Remington RD, Macdonald M: Joint study of extracranial arterial occlusion. V. Progress report of prognosis following surgery or nonsurgical treatment for transient cerebral ischemic attacks and cervical carotid artery lesions. J Am Med Assoc 1970;211:1993–2003.

3   Shaw DA, Venables GS, Cartlidge NEF, Bates D, Dickinson PH: Carotid endarterectomy in patients with transient cerebral ischemia. J Neurol Sci 1984;64:45–53.

4   Hankey GJ, Warlow CP, Sellar RJ: Cerebral angiographic risk in mild cerebrovascular disease. Stroke 1990;21:209–222.

5   Dion JE, Gates PC, Fox AJ, Barnett HJM, Blom RJ: Clinical events following neuro-angiography: A prospective study. Stroke 1987;18:997–1004.

6   European Carotid Surgery Trialists' Collaborative Group: MRC European Carotid Sur-

gery Trial: interim results for symptomatic patients with severe (70–99%) or with mild (0–29%) carotid stenosis. Lancet 1991;25:1235–1243.

7   North American Symptomatic Carotid Endarterectomy Trial Collaborators: Beneficial effect of carotid endarterectomy in symptomatic patients with high-grade carotid stenosis. N Engl J Med 1991;325:445–453.

8   Beebe HG, Clagett GP, DeWeese JA, Moore WS, Robertson JT, Sandok B, Wolf PhA: Assessing risk associated with carotid endarterectomy. A statement for health professionals by an ad hoc committee on carotid surgery standards of the Stroke Council, American Heart Association. Circulation 1989;79:472–473.

9   Millikan C, Futrell N: The fallacy of the lacune hypothesis. Stroke 1990;21:1251–1257.

10 Imparato AM, Riles TS, Mintzer R, Baumann FG: The importance of hemorrhage in the relationship between gross morphologic characteristics and cerebral symptoms in 376 carotid artery plaques. Ann Surg 1983;197:195–203.

11 Lennihan L, Kupsky WJ, Mohr JP, Hauser WA, Correll JW, Quest DO: Lack of association between carotid plaque hematoma and ischemic cerebral symptoms. Stroke 1987;18:879–881.

12 Kessler Ch, Reuther R, Berentelg J, Kimmig B: The clinical use of platelet scintigraphy with 111In-oxine. J Neurol 1983;229:255–261.

13 Henningsen H: Indium-111-Plättchenszintigraphie bei Schlaganfallpatienten; in Kessler Ch (ed): Plättchenfunktion und Gefäßwand. Bad Oeynhausen, TM Verlag, 1989.

14 Hennerici M, Steinke W: Untersuchungen zur Entwicklung extrakranieller Karotisplaques mit der farbkodierten Duplexsonographie; in Kessler Ch (ed): Plättchenfunktion und Gefässwand. Bad Oeynhausen, TM Verlag, 1989.

15 Eagle KA, Boucher CA: Cardiac risk of noncardiac surgery. N Engl J Med 1989;321:330–332.

16 Graor RA, Hetzer NR: Management of coexistent carotid artery and coronary artery disease. Stroke 1988;19:1441–1444.

17 Hennerici M, Hülsbömer H-B, Hefter H, Lammerts D, Rautenberg W: Natural history of asymptomatic extracranial arterial disease. Results of a long-term prospective study. Brain 1987;110:777–791.

18 Chambers BR, Norris JW: Outcome in patients with asymptomatic neck bruits. N Engl J Med 1986;315:860–865.

19 Moneta GL, Taylor DC, Nicholls StC, Bergelin RO, Zierler RE, Kazmers A, Clowes AW, Strandness DE Jr: Operative versus nonoperative management of asymptomatic high-grade internal carotid artery stenosis: Improved results with endarterectomy. Stroke 1987;18:1005–1010.

20 The CASANOVA Study Group: Carotid surgery versus medical therapy in asymptomatic carotid stenosis. Stroke 1991;22:1229–1235.

21 The Asymptomatic Carotid Atherosclerosis Study Group: Study design for randomized prospective trial of carotid endarterectomy for asymptomatic atherosclerosis. Stroke 1989;20:844–849.

22 Mayo Asymptomatic Carotid Endarterectomy Study Group: Effectiveness of carotid endarterectomy for asymptomatic carotid stenosis. Design of a clinical trial. Mayo Clin Proc 1989;64:897–904.

23 A Veterans Administration Cooperative Study: Role of carotid endarterectomy in asymptomatic carotid stenosis. Stroke 1986;17:534–539.

24   Kleiser B, Widder B: Course of carotid artery occlusions with impaired cerebrovascular reactivity. Stroke 1992;23:171–174.
25   Ricotta JJ: Carotid endarterectomy in patients with asymptomatic carotid stenosis; in Norris JW, Hachinski VC (eds): Prevention of Stroke. Berlin, Springer, 1991.
26   Hertzer NR, Loop FD, Beven EG, O'Hara PJ, Krajewski LP: Surgical staging for simultaneous coronary and carotid disease: A study including prospective randomization. J Vasc Surg 1989;9:455–463.

Prof. Dr. O. Busse
Chefarzt der Neurologischen Klinik
Klinikum Minden
Friedrichstraße 17
D-32427 Minden (FRG)

Dorndorf W, Marx P (eds): Stroke Prevention.
Basel, Karger, 1994, pp 144–152

Balloon Angioplasty

Martin M. Brown

Division of Clinical Neuroscience, St George's Hospital Medical School, London, UK

Despite many recent advances in the prevention of stroke, including the publication of the Carotid Surgery Trials, the ideal treatment which would prevent stroke from carotid stenosis without risk, remains to be developed. Percutaneous transluminal balloon angioplasty is a new technique that may provide an alternative to endarterectomy, and which may be especially appropriate for patients who are not fit for surgery. The concept of passing a catheter along arteries towards the heart was greeted with concern that the procedure was highly dangerous when it was first introduced in the 1920s, but invasive catheterization is now accepted without question in the management of cardiac patients. We are following 10 years behind in the footsteps of our cardiac colleagues, and similar anxieties are frequently expressed today about carotid angioplasty. However, there is considerable evidence to suggest that the procedure has an acceptable risk rate and may be an appropriate treatment for certain patients.

The first percutaneous treatment for atherosclerotic peripheral vascular stenosis was reported by Dotter and Judkins [1] in 1964. These authors used graduated co-axial Teflon catheters in a manner analogous to the treatment of oesophageal stricture. Four years later, Staple [2] introduced a tapering catheter which was less traumatic, but the real advance in technology which allowed today's developments was the introduction of inflatable balloon dilation catheters, again first used in peripheral arterial stenosis by Gruntzig and Hopff [3]. Coronary percutaneous transluminal angioplasty (PTA) was introduced in 1977 [4] and rapidly became a very popular option for the treatment of ischemic heart disease, and by 1986 over 150,000 were performed in the USA. At the same time there was a rapid improvement in techniques and balloon technology, with success rates for both peripheral and coronary PTA approaching 90% [5, 6].

It is important to consider the rates of embolization from PTA as this is the main concern about using PTA in the cerebral circulation. Indeed, a number of authorities have specifically rejected the use of PTA for cerebrovascular disease because of the risks of cerebral embolism. In one large series of coronary PTA, the rate of nonfatal myocardial infarction, which presumably reflects the risk of embolization, was 4% [5]. Similar distal embolization rates of 5% have been reported in peripheral vascular disease [6]. If similar embolization rates accompany PTA of the carotid arteries, the procedure will compare well with the conventional treatment of carotid stenosis, carotid endarterectomy.

Despite the undoubted value of carotid endarterectomy in preventing stroke, surgery carries significant risks at the time of operation. An early series reported the risks of major stroke or death following carotid surgery as high as 21% [7]. Fortunately, with improved techniques and careful patient selection, series in academic centres reported morbidity as low as 4% [8], or even 2% if highly selected patients were operated on in the very best centres [9]. We are now fortunate to have more generalizable figures from the two recently published large multicentre randomized trials. The European Carotid Surgery Trial (ECST) reported a risk of major stroke or death during surgery for severe carotid stenosis of 7.5%, while the North American Symptomatic Carotid Endarterectomy Trial (NASCET) reported a slightly better surgical risk of 5% [10, 11]. Apart from the risk of stroke, there are also anaesthetic risks, including myocardial infarction, particularly in patients with ischemic heart disease or severe hypertension, pneumonia, deep vein thrombosis and pulmonary embolism [9 , 12]. In addition, there may be morbidity from cranial nerve injury, usually hyperglossal and occasionally facial nerve palsy. There are also the minor complications of wound haematoma, infection and cutaneous nerve injury. A review of the surgical complications of carotid endarterectomy in the ECST (pp. 122–130, this volume) suggests that advances in technique are unlikely to improve these risks significantly. Some patients are not fit for surgery and in these patients the risks of PTA will need to be compared with medical treatment, which carried a risk of major stroke of 22% over 3 years in ECST and a risk of any stroke of 28% over 2 years in NASCET.

PTA has several major advantages. The procedure is performed under local anaesthetic avoiding an incision in the neck and the complications of general anaesthesia. Admission to hospital can be limited to 48 h, which is important in these days of financial stringency. One major advantage is that the procedure is suitable for patients in whom carotid surgery is contraindicated, such as patients with severe ischemic heart disease [13], patients with surgically inaccessible lesions (such as high internal carotid stenosis), fibromuscular dysplasia [14–16], or fibrotic re-stenosis after endarterectomy [17–19], which are very easily dilated by an angioplasty balloon.

These considerations led us to carry out a feasibility study of PTA for patients with internal carotid artery stenosis at the Royal London Hospital [13]. The two reasons for treating carotid stenosis are to remove a source for thromboembolism and to improve perfusion pressure as a protection against haemodynamic stroke. PTA might be better at achieving the latter than the former. Initially we therefore chose patients with features of haemodynamic ischemia, including transient ischemic attacks occurring during orthostasis and patients with severe bilateral carotid stenosis and diminished cerebrovascular reserve, measured by cerebral blood flow reactivity to carbon dioxide inhalation. By 1991, we had treated 12 patients who were all relatively young with a mean age of 56 years and a range of 46–66 years. Most of the patients also had contraindications to endarterectomy, including ischemic heart disease (5 patients), poorly controlled hypertension (1 patient), severe arthritis preventing flexion of the neck (2 patients) and high cervical fibromuscular dysplasia (1 patient). Our results confirmed that PTA was feasible. Using single balloon dilation catheters with an inflated balloon diameter of 5 mm and length of 5 cm, 10 arteries were successfully dilated in 8 of the patients. In 2 patients cannulation of the internal carotid artery failed for technical reasons, in 1 patient the internal carotid artery became occluded during the angiogram and in 2 patients the procedure was abandoned because of transient symptoms during attempted cannulation. Four patients also developed neurological deficits during successful balloon inflation, but all of these were transient, most recovering within a few minutes, and the longest recovering within 2 h. No patient suffered a stroke. More recently, we have treated a few more patients with presumed thromboembolic, rather than haemodynamic, symptoms from carotid stenosis with similar success rates and lack of serious complications.

Our results are similar to others published in the literature. I have managed to find reports of 142 patients who have had atheromatous internal carotid artery stenosis treated by PTA (table 1). Initially these

Table 1. Published reports of PTA for atheromatous internal carotid stenosis

Report	Patients, n	Transient complications	Minor stroke	Major stroke
Wiggli and Gratzl, 1983 [20]	2	0	0	0
Brockenheimer and Mathias, 1983 [21]	3	1	0	0
Tsai et al., 1986 [15]	6	0	0	0
Theron et al., 1987 [18]	5	0	0	0
Freitag et al., 1987 [22]	11	1	0	0
Mathias, 1987 [16]	15	2	0	0
Theron et al., 1990 [23]	13	0	0	0
Brown et al., 1991 (this report)	12	4	0	0
Kachel et al., 1991 [24]	35	2	0	0
Munari et al., 1991 [25]	40	2	3	1
Total	142	12	3	1

were small case reports, but recently Kachel et al. [24] from the former GDR, and Porta et al. [25] from Bergamo, Italy, have reported series with 35 and 40 patients, respectively. Transient complications have been reported in about 10% of these patients, but only 3 minor strokes and 1 major stroke have been reported to date.These results are encouraging and suggest that the procedure has a similar risk to that of carotid surgery. However, this data must be treated with caution as series with a high complication rate are much less likely to have been published.

Most groups have used single balloon dilation catheters, but it is worth considering the technique proposed by Theron et al. [23], designed to prevent cerebral embolism during angioplasty. This technique uses a triple co-axial catheter and an occlusive balloon, which is inflated in the carotid artery above the stenosis before angioplasty is performed. The angioplasty balloon is then positioned and inflated across the stenosis. After deflation and withdrawal of the angioplasty balloon, debris is aspirated from below the occlusive balloon before this is also deflated and withdrawn. Theron et al. [23] found cholesterol crystals in 4 out of the 6 patients in whom they examined this debris. There are a number of disadvantages of balloon occlusion, including difficulty placing the introducor catheter, the increased complexity of the procedure and a considerable prolongation in the total catheter time, which all increase the hazards of the procedure. In addition, the period of total internal carotid artery occlusion is 10 min or more, which seriously increases the risks of haemodynamic ischaemia. This contrasts with the maximum of 30 s of balloon inflation which we have used, and we therefore continue to prefer the more simple single balloon technique.

It is worth considering the mechanism of balloon angioplasty. One tends to imagine atheroma as a porridge-like material and it is therefore surprising to find that angioplasty does not result in compression, stretching or re-distribution of atherosclerotic plaque. Instead the increase in luminal diameter results from stretching the vessel wall and an increase in the outer diameter of the vessel [26–29]. Experimental and a few human studies showed that balloon angioplasty causes desquamation of the intima and superficial splits in atherosclerotic plaque. Retraction of the intima and distension of the media results in the permanent increase in diameter of the vessel. These splits in the plaque are frequently accompanied by dissection which is therefore a common sequel to PTA. Splits in the plaque can be visualized by contrast medium after carotid angioplasty. Fortunately, dissection is usually limited to the site of angioplasty and rarely causes symptoms.

There are a number of potential risks of PTA. The major concern is embolic stroke resulting from dislodgement of thrombus or plaque material during catheterization of the stenosis or balloon inflation. Stroke may also occur from haemodynamic impairment of perfusion during occlusion of the artery at the time of procedure. Most of the few strokes described to date seem to have occurred from delayed embolism resulting from thrombus formation on the damaged intima or atheromatous plaque. Pseudoaneurysms may form as a result of persistent dissection and we have encountered arterial spasm distal to the site of dilation caused by a reaction to the catheter tip. In our hands this has always been asymptomatic, but if necessary could be treated with papaverine. Brief pain in the neck may accompany balloon dilation, especially if overdilation occurs, and stimulation of the carotid sinus with bradycardia and temporary asystole have been described. Although the preliminary results of PTA are encouraging, there remains considerable uncertainty about the procedure. Technical questions, such as which type of catheter to use, the optimum inflation pressure, the duration of inflation and monitoring requirements are uncertain. Prevention of embolism is an important consideration and a wide variety of different anticoagulant procedures have been used, including warfarinization, pretreatment with aspirin or ticlopidine and full heparinization. Should we use single balloons or distal proximal occlusion catheters? The clinical indications for PTA are equally uncertain. Should patients with haemodynamic and embolic symptoms both be treated? Should patients with ulcers or calcified lesions be excluded? Should PTA be offered in patients fit or carotid surgery, or only if carotid endarterectomy is contraindicated? Should the procedure be limited to carotid arteries, or include vertebral stenosis? Stenosis at the origin of the vertebral arteries is certainly very easy to treat by PTA, but the benefits are uncertain [16, 24, 30]. It is imperative that these questions should be answered before PTA enters general use in cerebrovascular disease.

We have therefore set up a randomized prospective international multicentre study, as the Carotid and Vertebral Artery Transluminal Angioplasty Study (CAVATAS) to try and answer some of these questions. The first patient was randomized into the pilot phase of the study in March 1992. The primary aims of CAVATAS are to determine the risks and benefits of carotid and vertebral PTA and to compare these with surgical treatment or best medical treatment alone. The secondary aims are to validate the use of different guidewires and catheters, to identify risk factors such as calcified plaques and to determine the recurrence rate of stenosis. Patients fit for surgery will be randomized in equal numbers between surgery and PTA. Patients who are not fit for surgery because of medical risk factors, inaccessible stenosis or those who refuse surgery will be randomized in equal numbers between PTA and medical treatment. All patients, irrespective of randomization, will receive the best available medical treatment. The protocol allows for the inclusion of symptomatic and asymptomatic patients, if intervention is considered appropriate, for example in a patient with severe carotid stenosis who requires cardiac surgery. At this stage of the study we have left details of the technique and catheter design to the preference of individual radiologists. Participating centre requirements include a physician with an interest in cerebrovascular disease, a vascular surgeon with expertise in carotid endarterectomy if patients are randomized to surgery, and a radiologist who has had training in neuroradiology and some experience of peripheral angioplasty. To date, 34 centres throughout Europe have expressed an interest in carotid angioplasty. CAVATAS provides a unique opportunity to scientifically study a new interventional procedure before it is entered to general use. Hopefully, carotid and vertebral PTA will turn out to be a useful treatment.

Zusammenfassung

Ballonangioplastie

Die perkutane transluminale Angioplastie (PTA) hat sich in der Behandlung koronarer und peripherer Gefäßstenosen mit Behandlungserfolgen bis zu 90% durchgesetzt [N Engl J Med 1988;318:265–270, Br Med J 1986;293:1047–1048]. Für Stenosen der Arteria carotis interna liegen bisher nur wenige Fallberichte vor. In einer eigenen Serie von 12 Patienten mit Symptomen einer hämodynamisch bedingten Karotisinsuffizienz, die mittels eines Einfachballons von 5 mm Durchmesser und 5 cm Länge dilatiert wurde, konnten 10 Arterien bei 8 Patienten erfolgreich dilatiert werden. Bei 2 Patienten scheiterte die Katheterisierung an technischen Schwierigkeiten, bei 2 weiteren wurde die Prozedur wegen transienter Symptome während des Versuches der Katheterisierung abgebrochen, und bei einem Kranken ereignete sich ein Gefäßverschluß während der Angiographie. Von den erfolgreich dilatierten Patienten entwickelten 4 ein in spätestens 2 h vollständig reversibles neurologisches Defizit. Bei wenigen Patienten mit vermutlich thromboembolisch wirksamen Karotisstenosen konnten vergleichbare Ergebnisse erzielt werden. Bei 142 bisher in der Literatur veröffentlichten Fällen lag die Rate transienter neurologischer Komplikationen bei etwa 10%. Zusätzlich ereigneten sich 3 Hirninfarkte mit geringem bleibendem Defizit und ein schwerer Schlaganfall. Diese Komplikationsraten erlauben keinen Vergleich mit denen der Karotisendarteriektomie, da die Komplikationsrate der Angioplastie vermutlich dadurch zu niedrig eingeschätzt wird, daß besonders schlechte Ergebnisse nicht veröffentlicht werden. Der Erfolg der PTA beruht auf einer Retraktion der Intima und Dehnung der Media, während arteriosklerotische Plaques meist nur oberflächlich aufgespalten werden, was oft mit einer lokalen Gefäßwanddissektion verbunden ist. Die Risiken der PTA sind die Embolie atheromatösen oder thrombotischen Materials von der Stenose und hämodynamische Probleme während der Katheterisierung und Balloninflation. Die meisten bisher berichteten Schlaganfälle dürften jedoch auf Embolien von sekundär an der Dilatationsstelle durch die Intimaverletzung entstandenen Thromben zurückgehen. Pseudoaneurysmen und längere Gefäßwanddissektionen sind ebenso selten wie Gefäßspasmen. Offene Fragen der Angioplastie betreffen neben ihrer Komplikationsrate und Langzeitwirksamkeit auch technische Details. So ist z. Zt. nicht klar, ob Einzelballonkatheter dem zur Vermeidung von Embolien konstruierten Dreifachkoaxialkatheter [Am J Neuroradiol 1990;11:869–874] unter- oder überlegen sind.

Wegen der Unsicherheiten über die Wertigkeit der PTA ist eine prospektive internationale und multizentrische Studie, die Carotid and Vertebral Artery Transluminal Angioplasty Study (CAVATAS), begonnen worden. Primäre Ziele der Studie sind die Evaluation von Risiken und Nutzen der Methode, sekundäre Ziele die Prüfung verschiedener Führungsdrähte und Katheter, die Indentifikation von Risikofaktoren und die Stenoserezidivrate. Eingeschlossen werden symptomatische und asymptomatische Patienten. Die Randomisierung erfolgt zu gleichen Teilen zu PTA und Karotisendarteriektomie. Bei inoperablen Patienten (hohes Operationsrisiko, technisch nicht angehbare Stenose) wird mit medikamentöser Behandlung verglichen.

References

1   Dotter CT, Judkins MP: Transluminal treatment of arteriosclerotic obstruction: Description of a new technique and a preliminary report of its application. Circulation 1964;30:654–670.

2   Staple TW: Modified catheter for percutaneous transluminal treatment of arteriosclerotic obstructions. Radiology 1986;91:1041–1043.

3   Gruntzig A, Hopff H: Perkutane Rekanalisation chronischer arterieller Verschlüsse mit einem neuen Dilatationskatheter: Modifikation der Dotter-Technik. Dtsch Med Wochenschr 1974;99:2502–2510.

4   Gruntzig AR, Senning A, Seigenthaler WE: Non-operative dilation of coronary artery stenosis: Percutaneous transluminal coronary angioplasty. N Engl J Med 1979;301:61–68.

5   The National Heart, Lung and Blood Institute Registry: Percutaneous transluminal coronary angioplasty in 1985–86 and 1977–81. N Engl J Med 1988;318:265–270.

6   Campbell WB: Angioplasty for intermittent claudication. Br Med J 1986;293:1047–1048.

7   Easton JD, Sherman DG: Stroke and mortality rate in carotid endarterectomy: 228 consecutive operations. Stroke 1977;8:565–568.

8   Winslow CM, Solomon DH, Chassin MR, Kosecoff J, Merrick NJ, Brook RH: The appropriateness of carotid endarterectomy. N Engl J Med 1988;318:721–727.

9   Browse NL, Ross-Russel RW: Carotid endarterectomy and the Javid shunt: The early results of 215 consecutive operations for transient ischaemic attacks. Br J Surg 1984;71:53–57.

10 European Carotid Surgery Trialists Collaboration Group: MRC European Carotid Surgery Trial: Interim results for symptomatic patients with severe (70–90%) or with mild (0–29%) carotid stenosis. Lancet 1991;337:1235–1243.

11 North American Symptomatic Carotid Endarterectomy Trial Collaborations: Beneficial effect of carotid endarterectomy in symptomatic patients with high grade carotid stenosis. N Eng J Med 1991;325:445–453.

12 Sundt TM; Sandok BA, Whisnant JP: Carotid endarterectomy: Complications and preoperative assessment of risk. Mayo Clin Proc 1975;50:301–306.

13 Brown MM, Butler P, Gibbs J, Swash M, Waterston J: Feasibility of percutaneous transluminal angioplasty for carotid artery stenosis. J Neurol Neurosurg Psychiatry 1990;53:238–243.

14 Hasso AN, Bird CR, Zinke DE, Thompson JR: Fibromuscular dysplasia of the internal carotid artery: Percutaneous transluminal angioplasty. Am J Neuroradiol 1981;2:175–180.

15 Tsai FY, Matovich V, Hiesheima G, et al: Percutaneous transluminal angioplasty of the carotid artery. Am J Neuroradiol 1986;7:349–358.

16 Mathias K: Katheterbehandlung der arteriellen Verschlusskrankheit supraaortaler Gefässe. Radiologe 1987;27:547–554.

17 Tievsky AL, Druy EM, Mardiat JG: Transluminal angioplasty in post-surgical stenosis of the extracranial carotid artery. Am J Neuroradiol 1983;4:800–802.

18 Theron J, Raymond J, Cassasco A, Courthoux F: Percutaneous angioplasty of atherosclerotic and post-surgical stenosis of the carotid arteries. Am J Neuroradiol 1987;8:495–500.

19 Courtheoux P, Theron J, Tournade A, Maiza D, Henriet JP, Braun JP: Percutaneous endoluminal angioplasty of post-endarterectomy carotid stenosis. Neuroradiology 1987;29:186–189.

20 Wiggli U, Gratzl O: Transluminal angioplasty of stenotic carotid arteries – Case reports and protocol. Am J Neuroradiol 1983;4:793–795.

21 Brockenheimer SAM, Mathias K: Percutaneous transluminal angioplasty in arteriosclerotic internal carotid artery stenosis. Am J Neuroradiol 1983;4:791–792.

22 Freitag G, Freitag J, Koch R-D, Heinrich P, Wagemann W, Hennig H-P, Deike R: Transluminal angioplasty for the treatment of carotid artery stenosis. Vasa 1987;16:67–71.

23 Theron J, Courtheoux P, Alachkar F, Bouvard G, Maiza D: New triple coaxial catheter system for carotid angioplasty with cerebral protection. Am J Neuroradiol 1990;11:869–874.

24 Kachel R, Basche S, Heerklotz I, Grossmane K, Endler S: Percutaneous transluminal angioplasty of supra-aortic arteries, especially the internal carotid artery. Neuroradiology 1991;33:191–194.

25 Munari L, Porta M, Belloni G, Moschini L, Ubbiali A: Carotid percutaneous angioplasty: Technical notes and follow-up. Neurol Res, in press.

26 Castaneda-Zuniga WR, Formanek A, Tadavarthy M, et al: The mechanism of balloon angioplasty. Radiology 1980; 135:565–571.

27 Block PC, Fallon JT, Elmer D: Experimental angioplasty – Lessons from the laboratory. Am J Roentgenol 1980;135:907–912.

28 Block P, Myler RK, Stertzer S, Fallon JT: Morphology after transluminal angioplasty in human beings. N Engl J Med 1981;305:382–385.

29 Clouse ME, Tomaschefski JF, Reinhold RE, Costello P: The mechanical effect of balloon angioplasty. Case report with histology. Am J Roentgenol 1981;137:867–871.

30 Motarjeme A, Keifer JW, Zuska AJ: percutaneous transluminal angioplasty of the vertebral arteries. Radiology 1981;139:715–717.

Martin M. Brown, MD
Senior Lecturer in Neurology
St George's Hospital Medical School
University of London
London SW 17 (UK)

Cardioembolic Stroke

Dorndorf W, Marx P (eds): Stroke Prevention.
Basel, Karger, 1994, pp 153–164

Detection of Embolic Events by Ultrasound

M. Kaps

Department of Neurology, Justus Liebig University, Giessen, FRG

Embolic clots causing cerebral ischemia may originate from cardiac sources, ulcerative plaques (artery-to-artery embolism), and more seldom from the pulmonary veins. A clot descended from a peripheral venous thrombus may reach the cerebral arteries via right-to-left cardiac or pulmonary shunts (paradoxical embolism).

Diagnosis of embolic stroke is usually based on clinical and radiological features. Rapid onset, homonymous hemianopsia and isolated aphasia are considered to be typical clinical presentations. Association of cerebral and systemic embolism is very suggestive but unusual. Demonstration of a cardiac source and evidence of no other cause of stroke is diagnostically sufficient for practical purposes. In order to identify embolic stroke mechanisms, the main attempts were therefore hitherto directed on the detection of a cardiac source. However, many patients revealing cerebral emboli, diagnosed angiographically by isolated branch occlusions, lack adequate cardiac disease. Many infarcts in the territory of the deep perforating arteries are associated with an appropriate atherosclerotic stenosis as well as a potential cardiac source of embolism. On the other hand, potential cardiac source and cerebrovascular disease coexist in one third of the patients, impeding definite inferences regarding cause-effect relationship. For these reasons it is agreed that there is still a lack of reliable criteria conforming the embolic nature of stroke, which is likely to account to the high proportion of infarcts of unknown cause reported from stroke data banks.

Ultrasound investigations, namely continuous-wave (CW) Doppler sonography, proved to be very valuable for stroke classification detecting extracranial occlusive disease [2] and the extent of arteriosclerotic alteration of the carotid artery. However, little attention has been paid until now to a significant potential of ultrasound corroborating the embolic nature of stroke. Each ultrasound method may add specific information confirming an embolic nature of stroke. The purpose of this contribution is to describe signs of embolism, which can be depicted by duplex sonography, transcranial Doppler ultrasound (TCD) or most recently by transcranial color-coded sonography (TCSS) and Doppler monitoring systems.

Duplex Sonography

Duplex sonography is widely used for noninvasive detection of extracranial carotid disease. Carotid atherosclerosis as a *source* of arterio-arterial embolism has been studied extensively. Nevertheless, the significance of distinct atheromatous deposits is still controversial and assessment of the individual risk originating from different plaque morphologies remains doubtful. Compared with this, surprisingly little attention was directed on floating clots *entrapped* in the carotid artery, which is highly suggestive for an embolic nature of stroke.

Doppler blood flow imaging findings in embolic occlusion of the cervical carotid artery are demonstrated exemplarily in 2 patients:

Patient 1 (fig. 1) was admitted with a severe sensorimotor hemiparesis. Initial CW Doppler sonography examination disclosed common carotid occlusion, associated with thyreotoxic atrial fibrillation. Duplex sonography revealed a floating clot oscillating with cardiac action occluding the carotid lumen, but no underlying atheroma. Recanalization of the common carotid artery took place within 3 weeks leaving internal carotid occlusion and external carotid artery stenosis.

Patient 2 suffered weakness of the arm and motor aphasia with sudden onset. Internal carotid artery occlusion was found concomitant with non-rheumatic atrial fibrillation. Doppler blood flow imaging displayed a floating embolus 2 cm distal to the carotid bifurcation, which became adherent within 2 weeks, but compressibility was seen for more than 3 months. Recanalization did not occur in this case.

These case reports underline the value of Duplex sonographic examination in patients with cervical carotid artery occlusion associated with potential cardiac source for embolism. However, the arterial wall structures should be examined accurately, to rule out underlying atheroma, which may grow floating thrombi as well [1].

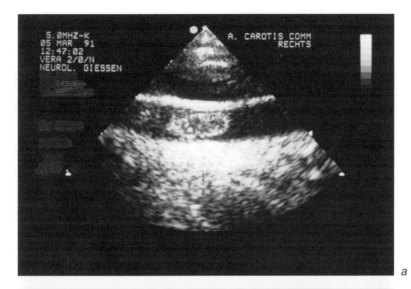

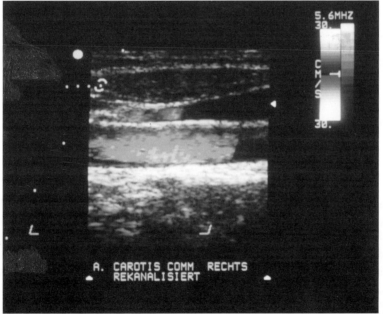

Fig. 1. Common carotid (CCA) occlusion in a 62-year-old patient with concomitant thyreotoxic atrial fibrillation. *a* Oval echogenic clot oscillates with cardiac action (5-MHz sector transducer). Arterial wall shows intact echo structure and no signs of underlying atherosclerosis. *b* Recanalization of the CCA 3 weeks later.

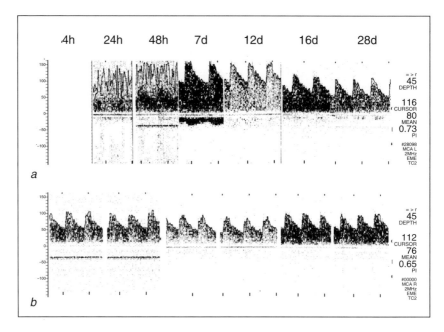

Fig. 2. 34-year-old patient suffering from cardiac embolism. *a* Recanalization of MCA beginning 24 h after clinical onset. Initially the stenotic signal is prominent; 28 days later the TCD signal is symmetric and normal on both sides. *b* Right MCA as reference.

Transcranial Doppler Ultrasound

Recanalization of occluded arteries in the vascular territory of the middle cerebral artery (MCA) is a typical feature of brain embolism. This phenomenon can be reliably diagnosed by TCD in patients with occlusion of the MCA main stem unfit for angiography during the acute phase of stroke (fig. 2). Serial TCD follow-up investigations carried out in 23 patients with MCA occlusions showed reperfusion in 16 cases [6]. In another TCD study comprising 22 patients with vanishing occlusions in the MCA territory, 20 cases met the criteria of cardioembolic stroke according to the NINDS classification [9]; 2 patients retained a residual MCA stenosis suggestive of atherosclerosis as the underlying cause [7].

Significant increase (side difference >25%) of blood flow velocity in initial TCD recordings during acute stroke is also most likely to represent postischemic hyperemia following recanalization [19]. This hyperemia is transient and normalizes within days (otherwise MCA stenosis must be taken into consideration). It must be emphasized therefore that TCD should be performed as early as possible after onset of suspected cerebral embolism and interpretation of the hemodynamic findings needs to be related in time to the ictal event. Under these prerequisites, TCD follow-up examinations may provide valid pathogenetic clues on embolic stroke.

Transcranial Color-Coded Sonography

Development of color Doppler imaging [10, 11] was the decisive step to TCCS, which allows imaging of basal cerebral arteries in the context of parenchymal structures. TCCS may overcome some key drawbacks of TCD, because it facilitates differentiation between basal arteries especially under pathological conditions and improves the accuracy and reproducibility of blood flow velocity measurements.

Figure 3 shows TCCS findings in a patient suffering from embolic MCA occlusion. Absent flow signal in the meningeal structures adjacent to the minor wing of the sphenoid and the Sylvian fissure where the MCA main stem is to be expected, is diagnostic for artery occlusion. Follow-up images of the affected arterial segment display the process of recanalization.

Further experience with TCCS in the near future will elucidate the impact of this new noninvasive bedside method on stroke classification and management.

TCD Monitoring

Very recently, automatic detection of arterial emboli using Doppler ultrasound has been introduced [13, 15, 18]. It is neither the source nor the recipient site of embolism, but the embolus itself that we are looking at. Emboli as they pass the probe cause Doppler signals of a much greater intensity than those reflected from blood cells. The amplitude of ultrasound power depends on the size and the acoustic impedance of particles carried in the bloodstream. This phenomenon has been observed in the cerebral circulation at first during cardiopulmonary bypass and carotid

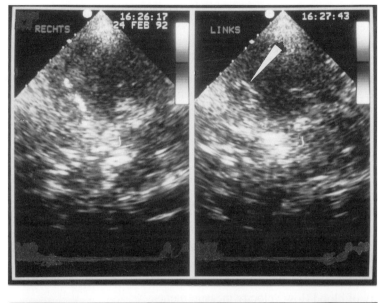

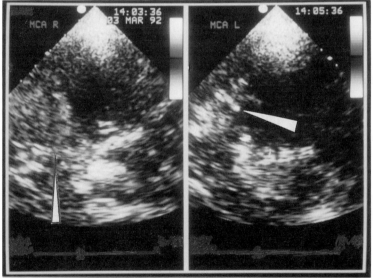

Fig. 3. TCCS displays recanalizing MCA occlusion. *a* Initial examination reveals normal right MCA. *b* Left MCA is occluded. Arrow points to meningeal structures of the Sylvian fissure, where the MCA would usually be expected. *c* Normal right MCA. ACA is coded blue (arrow), because blood flow is directed away from the probe. *d* Recanalization of the left MCA (arrow) was found 8 days later.

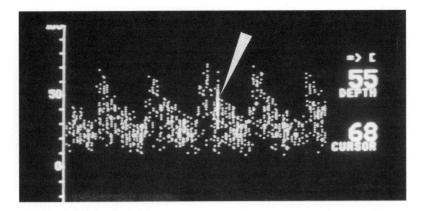

Fig. 4. 64-year-old patient with a prosthetic aortic valve. Doppler signal of high amplitude (arrow) caused by microembolization, which overloads the instrumentation and produces a characteristic 'chirping' sound.

endarterectomies [12, 17]. Recently, clinically silent microembolization was monitored in patients with prosthetic aortic valves [3] (fig. 4), patients suffering from amaurosis fugax [14] and stroke victims with history of atrial fibrillation [16].

These advances in Doppler monitoring technology open promising perspectives. Further studies in clinical setting will show its practicability and its impact on understanding stroke mechanism, on risk evaluation in subgroups and thus on primary and secondary prevention of stroke.

Echo Contrast Embolization

Detection of paradoxical cerebral echo contrast embolization by transcranial Doppler discovers a stroke mechanism which is worthy of being noted, especially in younger stroke victims and in patients with infarction of unexplained etiology. Clots from venous circulation may migrate into the systemic circulation in the presence of septal defects, pulmonary hypertension, Valsalva maneuver, AV fistula and hemorrhagic teleangiectasia.

Patent foramen ovale can be detected after injection of microcavitation contrast (generated by agitating a mixture of patient's blood, normal

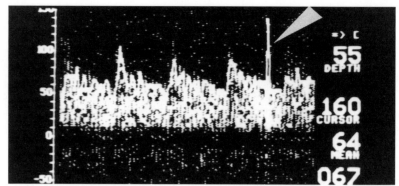

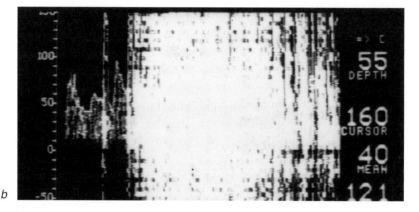

Fig. 5. 36-year-old patient with stroke of 'unexplained etiology'. *a* A single galactose particle (arrow) can be detected in the MCA after injection of echo contrast medium into the cubital vein. *b* Shower of echo contrast passes through the MCA immediately after release of Valsalva's maneuver.

saline and air) in the antecubital vein while monitoring MCA velocity signal. The results from these investigations suggest TCD as a sensitive technique for the detection of paradoxical embolism [4]. Transcranial contrast Doppler sonography using transesophageal echocardiography as reference method revealed a sensitivity of 87% and a specificity of 100% [8].

Our own experience (fig. 5) with echo contrast medium, which is a standardized suspension of soluble galactose particles (size <12 μm)

(Echovist®) indicates that the echo contrast test can be easily performed and is well tolerated by the patients. Serious side effects are not reported. However, patent foramen ovale can be detected in 34% of necropsies during the first three decades of life and is also frequent in the elderly (20–25%) [5]; the size of the defect increases with age (first decade: 3.4 mm; tenth decade: 5.8 mm). Accordingly, we found variable amounts of contrast medium trespassing from venous into the systemic circulation in stroke patients as well as in healthy volunteers. More extensive studies with strictly standardized methodology are therefore mandatory in order to assess the pathogenetic relevance of positive echo contrast tests and to establish a cause-effect relationship in individuals.

Conclusion

Currently available ultrasound techniques may add significant and reliable information about embolic stroke mechanisms. Subgroups carrying an increased risk of embolic stroke may be identified more precisely with monitoring systems which will have major impact on both primary and secondary prevention. These methods should therefore be used more extensively as a key to understand cerebral ischemic episodes.

Zusammenfassung

Ultraschalldiagnostik embolischer Schlaganfälle

Die Diagnose eines embolisch verursachten Schlaganfalls basiert üblicherweise auf klinischen und radiologischen Kriterien. Besondere Aufmerksamkeit wird außerdem dem Herzen als Ausgangspunkt kardiogener Hirnembolien zuteil. Trotzdem gibt es immer wieder Fälle, in denen es nicht gelingt, eine Emboliequelle zu finden. Andererseits existieren häufig auch konkurrierende Schlaganfallursachen. Methoden, die die Diagnose eines embolischen Hirninfarktes erhärten, sind daher von besonderem klinischem Interesse. Ultraschallverfahren sind nicht nur geeignet, arteriosklerotische Verschlußprozesse der extrakraniellen Hirnarterien als Ursache eines Schlaganfalles aufzudecken, sie können auch sehr verläßlich Hinweise für eine embolische Genese des Hirninfarktes liefern. Mit Hilfe der *Duplex-Sonographie* sind flottierende Thromben kardiogenen Ursprungs nachweisbar, die sich im Bereich der Karotisgabel verfangen. Wenn die Ultraschalluntersuchung unmittelbar nach Auftreten der klinischen Symptome durchgeführt wird, erkennt man thrombotisches Material, das synchron zum Pulsschlag flottiert. Später ist zu beobachten, wie das Gefäß rekanalisiert oder sich der Thrombus wandständig festhaftet. Charakteristisch ist, daß initial im Abschnitt des embolischen Gefäßverschlusses keine arteriosklerotischen Wandveränderungen erkennbar sind. Rekanalisierende Verschlüsse von Mediaästen gelten als verläßlicher Hinweis auf einen embolischen Hirninfarkt. Der Nachweis einer Rekanalisation des Mediahauptstammes kann mit Hilfe der *transkraniellen Doppler-Sonographie* (TCD) geführt werden. In einer TCD-Verlaufsstudie erfüllten 20 von 22 Patienten mit rekanalisierenden Verschlüssen im Strombahngebiet der Arteria cerebri media die Kriterien einer Hirnembolie nach der NINDS-Klassifikation [Stroke 1990;21:560–562]; 2 Patienten behielten nach Rekanalisation eine Stenose der A. cerebri media zurück als Hinweis auf eine arteriosklerotische Grundlage des akuten thrombotischen Mediaverschlusses [J Neurol 1992;239:138–142]. In einer anderen Serie von 23 Patienten mit akutem Mediaverschluß wurde in 16 Fällen eine Rekanalisation nachgewiesen [Stroke 1990;21:532–537]. Auch ein signifikanter Seitenunterschied der maximalen systolischen Strömungsgeschwindigkeit (mehr als 30%) als Ausdruck einer postischämischen Hyperämie kann unter bestimmten Voraussetzungen als Beleg dafür, daß eine Rekanalisation stattgefunden hat, gewertet werden. Da die intrakranielle Hämodynamik nach einem Schlaganfall sehr variabel ist und sich auch kurzfristig ändern kann, kommt es darauf an, daß transkraniell dopplersonographische Untersuchungen so früh wie möglich nach Eintritt der klinischen Symptome sowie im weiteren Verlauf durchgeführt werden.

Die *transkranielle Farb-Duplex-Sonographie* erlaubt eine Darstellung der basalen Hirnarterien vor dem Hintergrund der umgebenden Parenchymstrukturen. Es ist deswegen möglich, die Hirnarterien exakt zu lokalisieren und den Verschluß der A. cerebri media, der mit der konventionellen «blinden» TCD schwer zu beweisen ist, mit hoher Treffsicherheit zu diagnostizieren.

Kontinuierliche *Monitoringverfahren* erlauben den direkten Nachweis embolischer Ereignisse. Embolische Partikel erzeugen aufgrund eines starken Impedanzsprungs charakteristische Doppler-Signale von hoher Amplitude, wenn sie das Meßvolumen des Schallkegels passieren. Diese Phänomene sind bereits seit längerer Zeit bekannt und wurden u. a. während kardiopulmonaler Bypass-Operationen und Karotisendarteriektomien beobachtet [Transkranielle Doppler-Sonographie bei zerebrovaskulären Erkrankungen, Berlin, Springer, 1987, Anaesthesist 1988;37:256–260]. Mikroembolisationen wurden bei Patienten mit künstlichen Herzklappen [Proceedings of the 6th International Symposium on Intracranial Hemodynamics, San Diego, 1992], bei Patienten mit Amaurosis-fugax-Attacken [Transcranial Doppler, New York, Raven Press, 1992] und Patienten mit Vorhofflimmern [Proceedings of the 6th International Symposium on Intracranial Hemodynamics, San Diego, 1992] beschrieben. Inwieweit diese Verfahren zuverlässig genug sind, um das Risiko eines embolischen Hirninfarktes genauer einzuschätzen, muß in Zukunft durch weitere systematische Untersuchungen geprüft werden. Paradoxe Hirnembolien kommen durch Übertritt von embolischem Material aus dem venösen in das arterielle System zustande. Voraussetzung hierfür ist ein Rechts/Links-Shunt, der durch venös appliziertes *Echokontrastmittel* nachgewiesen werden kann. Transkraniell dopplersonographische Untersuchungen mit Echokontrastmittel und simultanem transösophagealem Echokardiogramm zeigen eine sehr hohe Übereinstimmung beider Methoden [7th International Symposium on Cerebral Hemodynamics, 1993]. Demnach gelingt auch der Nachweis eines offenen Foramen ovale mittels Echokontrastembolisation und TCD-Monitoring mit hoher Treffsicherheit. Es liegt nahe, daß sich mit Hilfe dieser Methode bei Patienten mit ungeklärter Ursache eines Schlaganfalls zusätzliche Informationen hinsichtlich der Ätiologie gewinnen lassen [65. Jahrestagung der Deutschen Gesellschaft für Neurologie, Saarbrücken, 1992]. Auch hier sind weitere systematische prospektive Untersuchungen notwendig, in denen parallel zur Echokontrastdiagnostik potentielle Ausgangspunkte venöser Thrombosen untersucht werden müssen.

References

1   Arning C, Herrmann HD: Floating thrombus in the internal carotid artery disclosed by B-mode ultrasonography. J Neurol 1988;235:425–427.

2   Bogousslavsky J, van Melle G, Regli: The Lausanne Stroke Registry: Analysis of 1000 consecutive patients with first stroke. Stroke 1988;19:1083–1092.

3   Berger M, Davis D, Lolley D, Rams J, Spencer M: Detection of subclinical microemboli in patients with prosthetic aortic valves. Proceedings of the 6th International Symposium on Intracranial Hemodynamics, San Diego 1992.

4   Chimowitz MI, Nemec JJ, Marwick TH, Lorig RJ, Firlan AJ, Salcedo EE: Transcranial Doppler ultrasound identifies patients with right-to-left cardiac or pulmonary shunts. Neurology 1991;41:1902–1904.

5   Hagen PT, Scholz DG, Edwards WD: Incidence and size of patent foramen ovale during the first 10 decades of life: An autopsy study of 965 normal hearts. Mayo Clin Proc 1984;59:17–20.

6   Kaps M, Damian MS, Teschendorf U, Dorndorf W: Transcranial Doppler ultrasound findings in middle cerebral artery occlusion. Stroke 1990;21:532–537.

7   Kaps M, Teschendorf U, Dorndorf W: Hemodynamic studies in early stroke. J Neurol 1992;239:138–142.

8   Karnik R, Stöllberger C, Valentin A, Winkler WB, Slany J: Detection of patent foramen ovale by transcranial contrast Doppler ultrasound. Cardiol 1992;69:560–562.

9   NINDS: Classification of cerebrovascular diseases. III. Stroke 1990;21:637–676.

10 Omoto R, Yokote Y, Takamoto S, et al: Clinical significance of newly developed real-time intracardiac two-dimensional blood flow imaging system (2-D Doppler). Jpn Circ J 1983;47:974.

11 Namegawa K, Kasai C, Koyano A: Imaging of blood flow using autocorrelation. Ultrason Med Biol 1982;8(suppl1):138.

12 Ries F, Eicke M: Auswirkungen der extrakorporalen Zirkulation auf die intrazerebrale Hämodynamik – Erklärung postoperativer neuropsychiatrischer Komplikationen? In Widder B (ed): Transkranielle Doppler-Sonographie bei zerebrovaskulären Erkrankungen. Berlin, Springer, 1987.

13 Russel D, Madden K, Clark WM, Sandset PM, Zivin JA: Detection of arterial emboli using Doppler ultrasound in rabbits. Stroke 1991;22:253–258.

14 Russel D: The detection of cerebral emboli using Doppler ultrasound; in Newell DW, Aaslid R (eds): Transcranial Doppler. New York, Raven Press, 1992, pp 207–213.

15 Spencer PS, Thomas GI, Nicholls SC, Sauvage LR: Detection of middle cerebral artery emboli during carotid endarterectomy using transcranial Doppler ultrasonography. Stroke 1990;3:415–423.

16 Tegeler H, Hitchings LP, Eicke M, Leighton J. Fredericks RK, Downes TR, Stump DA, Burke GL: Microemboli detection in stroke associated with atrial fibrillation. Proceedings of the 6th International Symposium on Intracranial Hemodynamics, San Diego 1992.

17 Thiel A, Russ W, Kaps M, Marck GP, Hempelmann G: Die transkranielle Dopplersonographie als intraoperatives Überwachungsverfahren. Anaesthesist 1988;37:256–260.

18   Klepper JR, Curry MA, Spencer MP: Automatic detection of cerebral emboli. Proceed-
      ings of the 6th International Symposium on Intracranial Hemodynamics, San Diego
      1992.
19   Zhu CZ, Norris JW: TCD – A new test for embolic stroke? Proceedings of the 6th
      International Symposium on Intracranial Hemodynamics, San Diego 1992.

PD Dr. M. Kaps
Neurologische Klinik
Justus-Liebig-Universität Giessen
Am Steg 14
D-35392 Giessen (FRG)

Dorndorf W, Marx P (eds): Stroke Prevention.
Basel, Karger, 1994, pp 165–179

Risk Evaluation of Anticoagulant Therapy in Cardioembolic Stroke

C. R. Hornig

Department of Neurology, Justus Liebig University, Giessen, FRG

Till today we have no controlled studies that enable a sufficient and reliable decision about the appropriate antithrombotic therapy for secondary prevention of cardioembolic stroke. Recommendations for anticoagulant therapy are mostly based on studies about primary prevention of thromboembolism in various cardiac diseases. Efficacy of oral anticoagulants is well proven for nonvalvular atrial fibrillation, ventricular thrombi remote from myocardial infarction, cardiomyopathy, and mechanical prosthetic cardiac valves. Heparin reduces the risk of thromboembolism after acute myocardial infarction significantly. No sufficient data are availabe for nonbacterial thrombotic endocarditis, infective endocarditis, patent foramen ovale, mitral valve prolapse, mitral annulus calcification, calcific aortic stenosis, atrial septal aneurysm, or heart tumors [10].

An effective regimen in primary prevention must not be the best choice for prophylaxis following cerebral ischemia. Patients with TIAs or ischemic strokes are at particular risk for bleeding complications due to anticoagulant therapy. Aggregate data of prospective randomized trials show that the probability of major hemorrhages is 2-fold higher for patients anticoagulated after a TIA or stroke than for those with myocardial infarction [39]. Therefore once cerebral ischemia had occurred, patients with certain underlying heart disaeses might perhaps make a larger profit from a less intense anticoagulant regimen or a platelet aggregation inhibitor. Even for mechanical prosthetic heart valves it has been shown that low-dose warfarin has the same prophylactic efficacy than higher doses, but significant less bleeding complications [57]. On the other hand, during the first 3 weeks after embolic brain infarction in several studies an increase of fibrinopeptide A and a decrease of antithrombin III has been reported, indicating an enhanced coagulation [14, 60, 62]. Therefore these patients might have a higher risk of thromboembolism requiring a more intensive anticoagulation.

Briefly, some basic questions concerning the optimal antithrombotic agent and its dosage for secondary prevention after cardioembolic stroke from different sources remain unanswered. Nevertheless, in many cases of cardioembolic stroke an agreement for anticoagulation exists. Different standpoints concern the begin of treatment: immediately within 48 hours, or late after 2 or 3 weeks.

Immediate Anticoagulation after Cardioembolic Stroke

Early anticoagulation after stroke means heparin or heparin followed by oral anticoagulants after some days. Neither therapeutic nor prophylactic efficacy of heparin after ischemic stroke has been proven yet. So it is not surprising that conflicting standpoints about its use can even be found among stroke specialists. On the one hand, no place is seen for heparin, as 'lack of benefit, a propensity to produce serious side effects, and procoagulant effects on platelet function make heparin an unattractive choice of therapy for patients with acute focal brain ischemia' [47]. On the other hand, it is practice to anticoagulate all patients with suspected or definite

Table 1. Immediate anticoagulation following cardioembolic stroke

Study	Patients		Cerebral recurrences		Hemorrhagic transformation	
	AC	CO	AC	CO	AC	CO
Furlan et al., 1982 [17]	25	29	2	5	1	0
Koller, 1982 [36]	15	29	0	4		
CESG, 1983 [9]	24	21	0	2	0	2
Hart et al., 1983 [24]	12	23	0	3		
Lodder and van der Luigt, 1983 [40]	21	18	2	0	2	
Calandre et al., 1984 [6]	25	17	1	0	4	3
Rothrock et al., 1989 [53]	49	72	1	1	3	5
Aggregate	171	209	3.5%	7.2%		

AC = Immediate anticoagulation; CO = late or no anticoagulation.

cardiogenic brain embolism immediately if no absolute contraindications exist [20]. About 60% of neurologists in the United States of America give heparin to more than 10% of their stroke patients within 24 h, predominantly to prevent recurrent cardioembolic stroke. But only 6% are convinced of its effectiveness [43].

Aggregate data of one prospective and several retrospective studies reveal a mean risk of early recurrent stroke of 7.2% for late or nonanticoagulated patients and of 3.5% for patients anticoagulated immediately after a cardioembolic stroke [6, 9, 17, 24, 36, 40, 53]. This difference is not statistically significant (table 1). Furthermore, if the risk of early recurrent embolism actually is about 7% and anticoagulation reduces the risk by 50%, 691 patients would be necessary in each treatment arm for a study with a type I error of 0.05 and a type II error of 0.2. The largest active treatment group of the available studies consisted of 49 patients only [53].

Therefore it is the only appropriate way now to evaluate the potential benefit and risk of heparinization in the individual case and then start anticoagulation immediately or with delay. Factors that have to be taken into account for risk evaluation are: reliability of diagnosis, risk of early recurrence, effectiveness of anticoagulants, risk of hemorrhagic infarction, risk of extracerebral bleeding, and risk of heparin-induced thrombocytopenia.

Reliability of Diagnosis

Risk evaluation of early anticoagulation must consider how definite the diagnosis of cardioembolic stroke is in the individual case. Due to intensive use of modern noninvasive or partly invasive diagnostic tools in many stroke patients, more than one possible etiology can be identified. In a series of 113 consecutive patients of our hospital with cerebral ischemia, all had extra- and transcranial Doppler ultrasound sonography, color-coded duplex sonography, transesophageal echocardiography and Holter electrocardiography. A potential source of cardiac embolism could be detected in 57 patients. One or more competitive reasons of stroke could be identified in about 74% of these patients. About 60% had an arteriosclerosis of the cerebral arteries, in most cases detected by ultrasound. A symptomatic stenosis or occlusion due to arteriosclerosis was found in 5 cases. 25% of the patients had evidence of a small vessel disease with hypertension or diabetes in history and multiple lacunes in CT or MRI.

How many of these patients with competitive etiologies actually had their stroke due to embolism from the heart or due to one of the other identified reasons, remains indefinite. Unfortunately there is a lack of sensitive and specific clinical criteria for a reliable diagnosis of a cardioembolic stroke [10, 49]. In many patients with a potential cardiac source of embolism the question whether the stroke actually was caused by embolism from the heart must therefore be left open. Immediate heparin anticoagulation of such a patient may be of no benefit or even harmful.

Early Recurrent Embolism

The risk of early recurrent embolism should not be overestimated. In 13 studies, 7.1% of 646 nonanticoagulated patients with a cardioembolic stroke experienced a recurrent cerebral ischemic event within 1–3 weeks; 6.3% of 223 patients suffered from noncerebral recurrent embolism, though the range of cerebral recurrences varied between 0 and 17% [3, 6, 9, 17, 24, 36, 40, 44, 53, 55, 56, 58, 60].

In a retrospective study of our own including 566 patients with a probable cardioembolic stroke, Kaplan-Meyer estimates revealed a lower recurrence rate of about 3% within 3 weeks after stroke (fig. 1).

The risk of embolism depends on the underlying heart disease, when looking at the primary event. It seems reasonable to suppose that this is also the case for recurrent embolism. Patients with an acute large myocardial infarction, infective endocarditis, rheumatic heart disease, or mechanical prosthetic heart valves are at higher risk than those with left ventricular aneurysm, nonvalvular atrial fibrillation, or mitral valve prolapse [10].

Certain factors are known to increase the risk of embolism. Patients with acute myocardial infarction are endangered if the infarct is large, transmural, located in the anterior wall, if a left ventricular thrombus has developed, or if a severe heart failure or atrial fibrillation has occurred [31].

Factors associated with an increased risk of thromboembolism in nonvalvular atrial fibrillation are age, left atrial thrombus, left atrial dilatation, left ventricular enlargement, previous myocardial infarction, high blood pressure, or spontaneous contrast echoes in the left atrium [1, 16, 22, 23, 27, 28, 42, 46, 54, 61, 66]. In a study of 272 patients with nonvalvular atrial fibrillation, three independent factors were found that increased the risk of embolism: left atrial size exceeding 4 cm, female gender, and

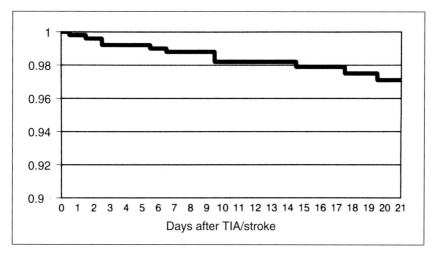

Fig. 1. Cumulative probability of survival without TIA or stroke after a cardiogenic brain embolism: n = 566, Kaplan-Meyer estimates; minor stroke (n = 3), major stroke (n = 3), fatal stroke (n = 2), TIA (n = 3).

structural heart disease. The probability of a thromboembolic event was 13 times higher if all three factors were present compared to only one [5]. It must be kept in mind that none of these paramenters have been proven as indicators of an increased risk of recurrent embolism after cardioembolic stroke. In a small series of 132 patients with ischemic stroke and nonvalvular atrial fibrillation, who were followed up for a mean of 5 years, risk factors for recurrent TIA or stroke were (odds ratio, 95% CI, p): initial epileptic seizures – 6.5, 1.8–23.1, 0.001; mild or moderate deficit – 2.8, 1.2–6.5, 0.011; hypertension – 2.4, 1.1–5.2, 0.028) [32].

Effectiveness of Anticoagulation

A crucial question concerning immediate anticoagulation is whether and to what extent a certain anticoagulant decreases the risk of recurrent embolism. Depending on the underlying cardiac disease a variety of embolic material has to be taken into account: red fibrin-dependent thrombi, white platelet-fibrin thrombi, noninfected valvular vegetations, infected valvular vegetations, calcific tissue and myxomatous debris. From the mode of action of heparin hardly any preventive effect is to be expected in the case of white platelet thrombi or calcific emboli. For many cardiac sources of embolism, heparin has not been proven to reduce thrombo-embolic complications. Wide experiences with heparin anticoagulation exist for acute myocardial infarction, after which the risk of a complicating stroke is reduced by about 50% [12, 26, 31, 52, 63, 64, 67].

Hemorrhagic Infarction

Frequency of hemorrhagic transformation of cerebral infarcts is lowest in retrospective CT studies and highest in autopsy series of acute embolic stroke (mean 58%) [15, 35]. Serial CT examinations revealed an incidence of 22–43%, as many of the bleedings occur not before the second week, when routine CTs are usually no longer performed [29, 38, 45]. Actually, hemorrhagic transformation may even be more frequent. Small amounts of blood may be not visible by CT. MRI is more sensitive and degradation products of blood are detectable for several weeks after

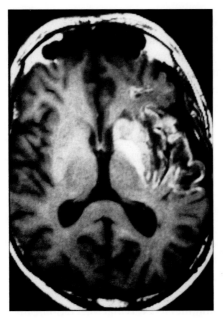

Fig. 2. Hemorrhagic transformation of a middle cerebral artery infarction due to cardiogenic brain embolism from left atrial thrombus (MRI, T1-weighted image, 3 weeks after stroke).

the bleeding. In a small series of 26 consecutive nonanticoagulated patients with middle cerebral artery infarction due to cardiogenic embolism, we found about 70% of the infarcts hemorrhagic in MRI 3 weeks after stroke. Hemorrhagic transformation was a regular finding if the infarction area exceeds 3 cm maximal diameter (fig. 2).

The first time a hemorrhage in brain infarcts of different etiology is visible in CT is predominantly the second (54%) or the first week (39%) after stroke. Infarcts due to cardiogenic embolism show a tendency to become hemorrhagic earlier, most of them within the first week [29].

Because secondary bleeding in embolic brain infarcts is common, the question could not be whether hemorrhagic transformation is more frequent under anticoagulation. The rather important question is whether anticoagulation results in more severe cerebral bleedings. Without therapeutic anticoagulation about 50% of secondary hemorrhages are petechial bleedings, predominantly in the cortex. They are visible by CT in the second or even third week after stroke. The underlying mechanism in many cases might be the restoration of circulation to the injured capillary bed by establishment of collateral circulation, when ischemic edema resolves. Small hematomas are predominantly seen within the basal ganglia probably due to confluent petechial hemorrhages and count for about 25% of all secondary hemorrhages. Confluent purpura within larger parts of the infarct (about 17%) appear rather hyperdense in CT. About 7% of all secondary hemorrhages in CT resemble massive intracerebral hemorrhages. The predominant mechanism of such severe bleeding is restoration of blood flow in a larger injured vessel by reopening of the initial side of occlusion [25, 29, 45].

Most hemorrhagic transformations are not associated with a clinical worsening. Only a few diffuse bleedings, certainly all large hematomas result in a clinical deterioration. Most anecdotal reports of hemorrhagic infarcts with clinical worsening deal with anticoagulated patients. In four larger reports of secondary hemorrhagic infarcts, the bleeding caused a clinical worsening in a mean of 19.6% of 51 anticoagulated patients compared to 9.8% of 112 nonanticoagualted [8, 29, 30, 38]. Therefore, there is some evidence, although no proof, that the common and in most cases clinically silent hemorrhagic transformation might be accentuated by anticoagulation with clinical deterioration.

Such massive intracerebral hemorrhages occur within the first days after stroke; about 60% of the patients do not survive. The mean interval between cerebral embolism and cerebral hematoma was 2.5 days (range

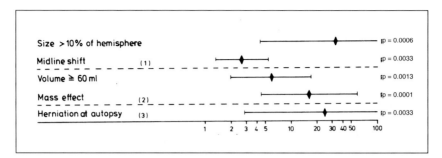

Fig. 3. Factors increasing the risk of hemorrhagic transformation of cerebral ischemic infarction (odds ratio, 95% CI): Data taken from: (1) Okada et al. [45], n = 65/95; (2) Hornig et al. [29], n = 28/27, and (3) Lodder et al. [41], n = 16/32 (number of hemorrhagic infarcts/number of nonhemorrhagic infarcts).

1–11 days) in 5 reports of altogether 24 patients, who were immediately anticoagulated with heparin after stroke. The interval between start of heparin prophylaxis and bleeding was 1.5 days (range 1–9 days). More than 50% of these patients with massive hemorrhages were hypertensive or had an excessive anticoagulation. By the way, a PTT ratio between 2.5 and 3 sometimes was interpreted as excessive. All patients had an at least medium-sized infarct [2, 7, 8, 11, 58].

The size of the cerebral infarct has been identified as the only predictor of its hemorrhagic transformation accordingly by different groups. The risk of bleeding is increased about 5-fold if the infarction volume exceeds 50 ml, and it is raised nearly 20-fold in the case of a mass effect (fig. 3) [29, 41, 45]. The prognostic significance of hypertension, age, or etiology of the infarct for hemorrhagic transformation is not definite yet.

Extracerebral Bleeding

The frequency of major bleeding complications of heparin therapy is well documented for venous thromboembolism. Analysis of an aggregate of 3,700 patient-days in prospective studies revealed a risk of 0.53%/day for a major hemorrhage [18, 33, 34]. In 8 prospective studies, 619 patients with cerebral ischemia of different causes were treated immediately with heparin anticoagulation. The target-PTT ratio varied between 1.5 and 3, the mean duration of treatment between 5 days and 3 weeks. A cerebral hematoma occurred in 1.5% of the patients, major extracerebral bleedings requiring interruption of anticoagulation or even transfusion in 3.7% [4, 9, 13, 21, 38, 48, 51, 59].

The risk of bleeding complications of heparin anticoagulation depends on the dose of heparin, the patient's anticoagulant response, the method of administration and some other patient-related factors. The influence of dose and patient's anticoagulant response can be controlled by monitoring the PTT. Nevertheless, practical experience teaches that it is difficult to achieve a rather constant PTT prolongation. Aggregate data of randomized studies revealed a risk of major hemorrhages of 11.8%, if heparin is given by intermittent intravenous injections, whereas only 5.3% of patients with continuous infusions developed major bleeding complications [39]. Patient-related factors of an increased risk of hemorrhages identified in two studies were female gender (×2), age about 60 years (×3), chronic alcohol consumption (×7), renal failure (×2), and comorbid conditions as serious cardiac illness, liver dysfunction, or a poor general condition (×2–5) [37, 65].

Heparin-Induced Thrombocytopenia

Two types of heparin-associated thrombocytopenia have to be differentiated [19]. The first type occurs soon after start of treatment and concerns 10% of all heparin-treated patients. Thrombocytopenia is the result of an enhanced platelet aggregation due to an inhibitory effect of heparin on thrombocyte adenylate cyclase. Platelet count seldom drops below 100,000/µl and normalizes within several days despite continuing heparin application.

Type II thrombocytopenia occurs 7–10 days after start of treatment. It may become manifest within a few hours if the patient has been exposed to heparin several times before. Frequency of this immunologically mediated type is estimated between 0.5 and 5%. Platelet count drops below 100,000/µl, often below 50,000/µl. Whereas the clinical relevance of type I heparin-induced thrombocytopenia is suspect, type II is associated with severe thromboembolic complications in about half of the cases.

In a prospective study about 5% of 137 patients with cerebral ischemia, who were anticoagulated with heparin, developed thrombocytopenia below 100,000/µl and about 15% had a platelet count drop by at least

40%. In the latter group the risk of extension of the brain infarct or a complicating myocardial infarction was increased 10-fold, probably due to a heparin-associated enhanced risk for thromboembolic events in the arterial bed [50].

Conclusions

Routine anticoagulation with heparin immediately after stroke due to a probable cardiogenic embolism does not seem to be justified, because: (a) the etiology of brain embolism is often not definite; (b) the risk of early recurrent embolism seems to be lower than assumed previously; (c) the efficacy of heparin has not been proven for many cardiac sources of embolism; (d) there is some evidence that hemorrhages into cerebral infarcts might be accentuated by heparin with clinical worsening; (e) a considerable risk of extracerebral major bleeding complications exists, and (f) there is a possible risk due to procoagulant effects of heparin on platelets.

Immediate anticoagulation for secondary prevention after cardioembolic stroke might be reasonable after risk evaluation considering: (a) the source of embolism in the heart; (b) factors associated with an increased risk of embolism; (c) the size of cerebral infarction; (d) the delay of treatment, and (e) factors associated with an increased risk of bleeding complications.

Zusammenfassung

Risikoabwägung der Antikoagulation nach kardioembolischem Schlaganfall

Die frühe Antikoagulation mit Heparin nach einem Schlaganfall zur Rezidivprophylaxe wird kontrovers diskutiert. In einer prospektiven und in 6 retrospektiven Untersuchungen liegt das durchschnittliche Risiko eines zerebralen Embolierezidivs innerhalb der ersten 2 bis 3 Wochen nach einer Hirnembolie bei 7,2% für spät oder nicht antikoagulierte Patienten und bei 3,5% für früh heparinisierte Kranke [Arch Neurol 1984;41:1152–1154; Stroke 1983;14:668–676; Neurology 1982;32:280–282; Neurology 1983;33:252–253; Neurology 1982; 32:283–285; Stroke 1983;14:42–46; Stroke 1989;20; 730–734]. Aufgrund der geringen Fallzahlen in diesen Untersuchungen ist dieser Unterschied statistisch aber nicht signifikant. Deshalb ist es geboten, vor einer eventuellen Frühheparinisierung in jedem Einzelfall eine Risikoabwägung vorzunehmen, in der berücksichtigt werden sollten: die Zuverlässigkeit der Diagnose einer Hirnembolie, das vermutliche Risiko eines frühen Embolierezidivs, die vermutliche Wirksamkeit einer Antikoagulation, das Risiko der Einblutung in einen Hirninfarkt, das Risiko extrazerebraler Blutungskomplikationen und die Gefahr einer heparininduzierten Thrombozytopenie.

Zuverlässigkeit der Diagnose: Von 113 konsekutiven Patienten mit zerebralen Insulten, die prospektiv mittels extra- und transkranieller Dopplersonographie, farbkodierter Duplexsonographie, transösophagealer Echokardiographie und Langzeit-EKG untersucht wurden, hatten 57 eine potentielle kardiale Emboliequelle. Von diesen hatten wiederum 74% eine weitere konkurrierende mögliche Ursache, meistens eine zerebrale Arteriosklerose. Da ausreichend sensitive und spezifische Kriterien für die Diagnose eines kardioembolischen Schlaganfalles fehlen, bleibt bei einer Reihe von Schlaganfallpatienten mit einer Embolie-quelle im Herzen die Frage offen, ob der Insult tatsächlich Folge einer kardiogenen Embolie oder nicht einer konkurrierenden Ursache gewesen ist.

Frühe Embolierezidive: In 13 Untersuchungen über Patienten mit kardioembolischem Schlaganfall bekamen 7,1% von 646 nicht antikoagulierten Patienten innerhalb von 1–3 Wochen einen erneuten zerebralen Insult, 6,3% von 223 Kranken erlitten eine systematische Embolie, wobei die Rezidivrate zwischen 0 und 17% variierte [Can J Neurol Sci 1983;10:32–36; Arch Neurol 1984;41:1112–1116; Stroke 1983;14:668–676; Neurology 1982;32:280–282; Neurology 1983;33:252–253; Neurology 1982;32:283–285; Stroke 1983;14:42–46; Acta Neurol Scand 1986;73:520; Stroke 1989;20:730–734; Stroke 1983;14:537–540; Neurology 1983;33:1104; Stroke 1984;15:426–437; Stroke 1991;22:12–16]. In einer eigenen Untersuchung, die 566 Patienten mit einem möglichen kardioembolischen Schlaganfall umfaßte, ergab die Kaplan-Meier-Statistik eine kumulative Rate zerebraler Rezidive von etwa 3% innerhalb von 3 Wochen. Das Rezidivrisiko wird im wesentlichen determiniert durch die zugrunde liegende Herzkrankheit und den aktuellen kardiologischen Befund.

Prophylaktische Wirksamkeit der Antikoagulation: In Abhängigkeit von der jeweiligen Herzkrankheit ist eine Vielzahl von embolischem Material in Betracht zu ziehen. Aufgrund der Wirkungsweise von Heparin ist nicht in jedem Fall ein präventiver Effekt zu erwarten und entsprechend ist für eine Reihe von Herzkrankheiten ein prophylaktischer Effekt von Heparin bisher auch nicht nachgewiesen worden.

Hämorrhagische Hirninfarkte: In Untersuchungsreihen mit seriellen computertomographischen Abteilungen beträgt die Inzidenz von Blutungen in Hirninfarkte 22–43%. In einer Serie von 26 konsekutiven nicht antikoagulierten Patienten mit A.-cerebri-media-Infarkten aufgrund einer kardiogenen Hirnembolie konnte mittels der sensitiveren Magnetresonanz-tomographie sogar in 70% der Infarkte 3 Wochen nach dem Schlaganfall Blut nachgewiesen werden. Infarkte mit einem Durchmesser über 3 cm zeigten regelmäßig Einblutungen. Die meisten hämorrhagischen Transformationen bleiben ohne klinische Folgen. Es ist zu vermuten, daß klinisch relevante Blutungen unter Antikoagulantien häufiger auftreten. In 4 größeren Untersuchungsreihen über sekundär hämorrhagische Hirninfarkte kam es durch die Blutung zu einer klinischen Verschlechterung bei durchschnittlich 19,6% von 51 antikoagulierten Patienten, verglichen mit 9,8% von 112 nicht antikoagulierten Kranken [Stroke 1984;15:779–789; Stroke 1986;17:179–185; Nervenarzt 1983;54:406–412; Nervenarzt 1991; 62:470–476]. Das Risiko schwerer Blutungen ist in der ersten Woche nach dem Schlaganfall am größten.

Extrazerebrale Blutungskomplikationen: Das Risiko schwerer extrazerebraler Blutungs-komplikationen wurde in 8 prospektiven Untersuchungen analysiert, die 619 Patienten mit ischämischen zerebralen Insulten unterschiedlicher Ätiologie umfaßten. Es betrug 3,7% innerhalb von 5 Tagen bis 3 Wochen [Stroke 1989;20:441–447; Stroke 1983;14:668–676;

Ann Intern Med 1986;105:825–828; Stroke 1987;19:10–14; Nervenarzt 1991;62:470–476; Arch Neurol 1985;42:960–962; Neurology 1984;34:736–740; Stroke 1990;21:1657–1662]. Ein erhöhtes Blutungsrisiko besteht für Frauen, ältere Patienten, chronische Alkoholiker und Kranke mit Niereninsuffizienz.

Heparininduzierte Thrombozytopenie: Die Häufigkeit des immunologisch vermittelten klinisch relevanten Typs 2 der heparininduzierten Thrombozytopenie wird zwischen 0,5 und 5% geschätzt, wobei es bei etwa der Hälfte der Betroffenen zu thromboembolischen Komplikationen kommen kann.

Schlußfolgerungen: Eine routinemäßige Antikoagulation mit Heparin unmittelbar nach einem kardioembolischen Schlaganfall erscheint derzeit nicht gerechtfertigt. Vielmehr ist im Einzelfall eine Risikoabwägung vorzunehmen unter Berücksichtigung der kardialen Emboliequelle, von Faktoren, die mit einem erhöhten Embolicrisiko einhergehen, der Größe des zerebralen Infarktes und von Faktoren, die mit einer erhöhten Gefährdung durch extrazerebrale Blutungskomplikationen verbunden sind.

References

1   Aronow WS, Gutstein H, Hsieh FY: Risk factors for thromboembolic stroke in elderly patients with chronic atrial fibrillation. Am J Cardiol 1989;63:366–367.
2   Babikian VL, Kase CS, Pessin MS, Norrving B, Gorelick PB: Intracerebral hemorrhage in stroke patients anitcoagulated with heparin. Stroke 1989;20:1500–1503.
3   Bass E: Anticoagulation in cerebral embolism. Can J Neurol Sci 1983;10:32–36.
4   Biller J, Bruno A, Adams HP Jr, Godersky JC, Loftus CM, Mitchell VL, Banwart KJ, Jones MP: A randomized trial of aspirin or heparin in hospitalized patients with recent transient ischemic attacks: A Pilot study. Stroke 1989;20:441–447.
5   Cabin HS, Clubb KS, Hall C, Perlmutter RA, Feinstein AR: Risk for systemic embolization of atrial fibrillation without mitral stenosis. Am J Cardiol 1990;65:1112–1116.
6   Calandre L, Ortega JF, Bermejo F: Anticoagulation and hemorrhagic infarction in cerebral embolism secondary to rheumatic heart disease. Arch Neurol 1984;41:1152–1154.
7   Cerebral Embolism Study Group: Cardioembolic stroke, early anticoagulation, and brain hemorrhage. Arch Intern Med 1987;147:636–640.
8   Cerebral Embolism Study Group: Immediate anticoagulation of embolic stroke: Brain hemorrhage and management options. Stroke 1984;15:779–789.
9   Cerebral Embolism Study Group: Immediate anticoagulation of embolic stroke: A randomized trial. Stroke 1983;14:668–676.
10 Cerebral Embolism Task Force: Cardiogenic brain embolism: The second report of the Cerebral Embolism Task Force. Arch Neurol 1989;46:727–743.
11 Drake ME, Shin C: Conversion of ischemic to hemorrhagic infarction by anticoagulant administration. Arch Neurol 1983;40:44–46.
12 Drapkin A, Merskey C: Anticoagulant therapy after acute myocardial infarction: Relation of therapeutic benefit to patient's age, sex and severity of infarction. J Am Med Assoc 1972;222:541–549.
13 Duke RJ, Block RF, Turpie AG, Trebilcock R, Bayer N. Intravenous heparin for the prevention of stroke progression in acute partial stable stroke: A randomized controlled trial. Ann Intern Med 1986;105:825–828.

14   Feinberg WM, Bruck DC, Ring ME, Corrgan JJ Jr: Hemostatic markers in acute stroke.
      Stroke 1989;20:592–597.
15   Fisher CM, Adams RD: Observations on brain embolism with special reference to the
      mechanism of hemorrhagic infarction. J Neuropathol Exp Neurol 1951;10:92–94.
16   Flegel KM, Shipley MJ, Rose G: Risk of stroke on nonrheumatic atrial fibrillation.
      Lancet 1987;i:526–529.
17   Furlan AJ, Cavalier SJ, Hobbs RE, Weinstein MA, Modic MT: Hemorrhage and anti
      coagulation after non-septic embolic brain infarction. Neurology 1982;32:280–282.
18   Gallus A, Jackaman J, Tillett J, Mills W, Wycherley A: Safety and efficacy of warfarin
      started early after submassive venous thrombosis or pulmonary embolism. Lancet
      1986;ii:1293–1296.
19   Greinacher A, Mueller-Eckhardt C: Diagnostik der Heparin-assoziierten Thrombo-
      zytopenie. Dtsch Med Wochenschr 1991;116:1479–1482.
20   Hacke W: Frühe Antikoagulation beim akuten ischämischen Hirninfarkt. Nervenarzt
      1991;62:467–469.
21   Haley EC, Kassell NF, Torner JC: Failure of heparin to prevent progression in progres-
      sing ischemic infarction. Stroke 1987;19:10–14.
22   Hall CA, Clubb S, Cabin HS: Atrial fibrillation and systemic embolization: Left atrial
      size strongly predicts risk of embolization in patients without mitral stenosis. J Am Coll
      Cardiol 1987;9:220A.
23   Halperin JL, Robert GH: Atrial fibrillation and stroke: New ideas, persisting dilemmas.
      Stroke 1988;19:937–941.
24   Hart RG, Coull BM, Miller VT: Anticoagulation and embolic infarction. Neurology
      1983;33:252–253.
25   Hart RG, Easton JD: Hemorrhagic infarcts. Stroke 1986;17:586–589.
26   Hilden T, Raaschou F, Iversen K, Schwartz M: Anticoagulants in acute myocardial
      infarction. Lancet 1961;i:327–331.
27   Hinton RC, Kistler JP, Fallon JT, Friedlich AL, Fisher CM: Influence of etiology of
      atrial fibrillation on incidence of systemic embolism. Am J Cardiol 1977;40:
      509–513.
28   Hirabayshi T: A study on the relationship between spontaneous contrast echoes in left
      atrium and cerebral embolism in patients with chronic atrial fibrillation by using
      transesophageal echocardiography. Hokkaido Ignaku Zassho 1991;66:179–186.
29   Hornig CR, Dorndorf W, Agnoli AL: Hemorrhagic cerebral infarction – A prospective
      study. Stroke 1986;17:179–185.
30   Hornig CR, Dorndorf W: Hämorrhagische Hirninfarkte – Klinik, computertomo-
      graphische Befunde, Progenose. Nervenarzt 1983;54:406–412.
31   Hornig CR, Kramer W, Dorndorf W: Hirnembolien nach Herzinfarkten. Akt Neurol
      1990;17:1–11.
32   Hornig CR, Will R, Dorndorf W: Ischämische zerebrale Insulte bei Vorhofflimmern:
      Eine retrospektive Untersuchung. Akteur Neurol 1989;16:195–200.
33   Hull RD, Raskob GE, Hirsh J: Continuous intravenous heparin compared with inter-
      mittent subcutaneous heparin in the initial treatment of proximal-vein thrombosis.
      N Engl J Med 1972;287:324–327.
34   Hull RD, Raskob GE, Rosenbloom D: Heparin for 5 days as compared with 10 days in
      the initial treatment of proximal venous thrombosis. N Engl J Med 1990;322: 1260–
      1264.

35 Jörgensen L, Torvik A: Ischemic cerebrovascular diseases in an autopsy series. 2. Prevalence, location, pathogenesis, and clinical course of cerebral infarct. J Neurol Sci 1969;9:285–320.

36 Koller RL: Recurrent embolic cerebral infarction and anticoagulation. Neurology 1982;32:283–285.

37 Landefeld CS, Cook EF, Flatley M, Weisberg M, Goldman L: Identification and preliminary validation of predictors of major bleeding in hospitalized patients starting anticoagulant therapy. Am J Med 1987;82:703–713.

38 Leonhardt C, Weiller C, Müllges W, Korbmacher G, Ringelstein EB: Antikoagulation beim akuten Schlaganfall: Nutzen, Risiken, Therapieversager. Nervenarzt 1991;62:470–476.

39 Levine MN, Hirsh J: Hemorrhagic complications of anticoagulant therapy. Semin Thromb Hemost 1986;12:39–57.

40 Lodder J, van der Luigt PJM: Evaluation of the risk of immediate anticoagulant treatment in patients with embolic stroke of cardiac origin. Stroke 1983;14:42–46.

41 Lodder J, Krijne-Kubat B, Broekman J: Cerebral hemorrhagic infarction at autopsy: Cardiac embolism and the relationship to the cause of death. Stroke 1986;17:626–629.

42 Maisch B, Grimm W, Langenfeld H, Elert O, Eigel P, Kochsiek K: Komplikationen der Herzschrittmachertherapie. Herzschrittmacher 1987;7:141–145.

43 Marsh EE III, Adams HP Jr, Biller J, Wasek P, Banwart K, Mitchell V, Woolson R: use of antithrombotic drugs in the treatment of acute ischemic stroke: A survey of neurologists in practice in the United States. Neurology 1989;38:1631–1634.

44 Norrving B, Nilsson B: Cerebral embolism of cardiac origin: The limited possibilities of secondary prevention. Acta Neurol Scand 1986;73:520.

45 Okada Y, Yamaguchi T, Minematsu K, Miyashita T, Sawada T, Sadoshima S, Fujishima M, Omae T: Hemorrhagic transformation in cerebral embolism. Stroke 1989;20:598–603.

46 Petersen P, Kastrup J, Helweg-Larsen S, Boysen G, Godtfredsen J: Risk factors for thromboembolic complications in chronic atrial fibrillation: The Copenhagen AFASAK study. Arch Intern Med 1990;150:819–821.

47 Phillips SJ: An alternative view of heparin anticoagulation in acute focal brain ischemia. Stroke 1989;20:295–298.

48 Putman SF, Adams HP Jr: Usefulness of heparin in initial management of patients with recent transient ischemic attacks. Arch Neurol 1985;42:960–962.

49 Ramirez-Lassepas M, Cipolle RJ, Bjork RJ, Kowitz J, Snyder BD, Weber JC, Stein SD: Can embolic stroke be diagnosed on the basis of neurologic clinical criteria. Arch Neurol 1987;44:87–89.

50 Ramirez-Lassepas M, Cipolle RJ, Rodvold KA, Seifert RD, Strand L, Taddeini L, Cusulos M: Heparin-induced thrombocytopenia in patients with cerebrovascular ischemic disease. Neurology 1984;34:736–740.

51 Ramirez-Lassepas M, Quinones MR, Nino HH: Treatment of acute ischemic stroke: Open trial with continuous intravenous heparinization. Arch Neurol 1986;43:386–390.

52 Report of the Working Party on Anticoagulant Therapy and Coronary Thrombosis to the Medical Research Council: Assessment of short-term anticoagulant adiminstration after cardiac infarction. Br Med J 1969;i:335–342.

53 Rothrock JF, Dittrich HC, McAllen S, Taft BJ, Lyden PD: Acute anticoagulation following cardioembolic stroke. Stroke 1989;20:730–734.

54   Ruocco NA, Most AS: Clinical and echocardiographic risk factors for systemic embolization in patients with atrial fibrillation in the absence of mitral stenosis. J Am Coll Cardiol 1986;7:165A.

55   Sage JI, van Uitert RL: Risk of recurrent stroke in patients with atrial fibrillation and non-valvular heart disease. Stroke 1983;14:537–540.

56   Santamaria J, Graus F, Peres J: Cerebral embolism and anticoagulation. Neurology 1983;33:1104.

57   Saour JN, Sieck JO, Mamo LAR, Gallus AS: Trial of different intensities of anticoagulation in patients with prosthetic heart valves. N Engl J Med 1990; 322:428–432.

58   Shields RW Jr, Laureno R, Lachman T, Victor M: Anticoagulant-related hemorrhage in acute cerebral embolism. Stroke 1984;15:426–437.

59   Slivka A, Levy D: Natural history of progressive ischemic stroke in a population treated with heparin. Stroke 1990;21:1657–1662.

60   Takano K, Yamagucki T, Kato H, Omae T: Activation of coagulation in acute cardioembolic stroke. Stroke 1991;22:12–16.

61   Tegeler CH, Hart RG: Atrial size, atrial fibrillation and stroke. Ann Neurol 1987;21:315–316.

62   Tohgi H, Kawashima M, Tamura K, Suzuki H: Coagulation-fibrinolysis abnormalities in acute and chronic phases of cerebral thrombosis and embolism. Stroke 1990;21:1663–1667.

63   Turpie A, Robinson JG, Doyle DJ: Comparison of high-dose with low-dose subcutaneous heparin to prevent left ventricular mural thrombosis in patients with acute transmural anterior myocardial infarction. N Engl J Med 1989;320:352–357.

64   Veterans Cooperative Study: Anticoagulants in acute myocardial infarction: Results of a cooperative clinical trial. J Am Med Assoc 1973;225:724–729.

65   Walker AM, Jick H: Predictors of bleeding during heparin therapy. J Am Med Assoc 1980;244:1209–1212.

66   Wiener I: Clinical and echocardiographic correlates of systemic embolization in non-rheumatic atrial fibrillation. Am J Cardiol 1987;59:177.

67   Wright IS, Marple CD, Beck DF: Report of the committee for the evaluation of anticoagulants in the treatment of coronary thrombosis with myocardial infarction. Am Heart J 1948;36:801–815.

PD Dr. Claus R. Hornig
Neurologische Klinik
Justus-Liebig-Universität Giessen
Am Steg 14
D-35392 Giessen (FRG)

Dorndorf W, Marx P (eds): Stroke Prevention.
Basel, Karger, 1994, pp 180–187

Nonvalvular Atrial Fibrillation and Stroke

P. J. Koudstaal

Department of Neurology, University Hospital Dijkzigt, Rotterdam, The Netherlands

'To this variety of apoplexy those are most liable who lead an idle life, who are obese, whose face and hands are constantly livid and whose pulse constantly unequal'

Wepfer, 1658

Atrial fibrillation (AF) is a common dysrhythmia, affecting 2–5% of the general population over the age of 60 [1–3]. It is found in about 15% of all stroke patients [4, 5], and in about 2–8% of transient ischemic attack (TIA) patients [6–8]. Causes of AF are atherosclerosis, rheumatic heart disease (RHD), hypertension, hyperthyroidism, cor pulmonale, and syphilis. The incidence of ischemic stroke in AF patients without RHD, so-called nonvalvular atrial fibrillation (NVAF), ranges between 2 and 5%/year [5, 9, 11]. In patients in whom no obvious cause of the AF can be found, so-called 'lone AF', the risk of embolism is substantially lower, ranging between 0.4 and 1%/year. Following an initial embolism, recurrent embolic events are most frequently observed during the first year [4, 10, 12, 13] and more specifically during the first 2 weeks. The stroke recurrence rate varies in different studies between 2 and 15% in the first year following the initial embolic event, and 5% yearly thereafter, and the mortality rate 5% yearly [4, 14]. The risk of recurrence is dependent on the type of cardiac abnormality [14]. Patients with combined RHD and AF show the highest recurrence rate [14]. The incidence of RHD, however, has strongly declined during the past years. Today, the most common cardioembolic source is NVAF [14]. Recent studies have shown that in NVAF patients without recent TIA or stroke, anticoagulants reduce the risk of embolic complications by two-thirds (primary prevention) [15–18]. Treatment with aspirin also lowers the risk [15, 16], but the exact size of the preventive effect still has to be established. The value of both anti-coagulation and aspirin in NVAF patients with a recent TIA or stroke (secondary prevention) is still unknown.

Is AF an Independent Risk Factor for Stroke?

It is evident that in some stroke patients the presence of AF is just coincidental, the dysrhythmia being merely a marker of advanced athero-sclerosis. The relationship might even be the other way round, that is, AF may be caused by the stroke. However, a causal relationship between AF and cerebral ischemic episodes is supported by both direct and indirect evidence: (1) there is a distinct clustering of ischemic episodes around the time of onset of AF [14, 19]; (2) the embolism rate may reach 30% in pa-tients with thyrotoxic atrial fibrillation [14]; (3) autopsy data from 56 pa-tients with a carotid occlusion showed that 11 were due to embolism from the heart (6 with combined AF and mitral stenosis and 2 patients with NVAF) [19]; (4) epidemiological data from the Framingham Study indi-cate that patients with NVAF have a 4-fold risk of stroke but no increased risk of developing ischemic heart disease [20]; (5) autopsy and angiogra-phical studies have shown that the fraction of strokes due to cardiogenic embolism in patients with NVAF ranges from 50 to 71% [21, 22] and (6) data from the Oxfordshire Community Stroke Project have shown a strikingly low prevalence of AF in patients with lacunar infarcts, which are supposed to be caused by small vessel disease and only in rare cases by embolism. Furthermore, new cardiological imaging techniques, such as transesophageal echocardiography and ultrafast CT, have been shown to be more accurate in the detection of intracardiac abnormalities than conventional techniques. Thus, one may conclude that NVAF, unassoci-ated with other cardiac or cerebrovascular disease, predisposes to cerebral embolism and that at least 60% (50–70%) of strokes in patients with NVAF are due to emboli from the heart [23].

Which Fibrillating Patients Have an Increased Risk of Cerebral Embolism?

Recent studies have identified the following risk factors for embolic complication: female sex; age; intermittent versus chronic AF; left atrial size; systolic hypertension; diastolic hypertension; prior myocardial infarct; angina pectoris; history of hypertension; congestive heart failure, prior thromboembolism [10, 24–28].

The majority of these risk factors were identified in a single study only. The reasons for discrepancies between studies are: (1) the definition of variables; (2) the study design, in particular the number and definition of major outcome events, and the duration of follow-up; (3) the antithrombotic therapy studied; (4) the statistical methods, in particular the use of a multivariate analysis, and (5) the number and type of variables studied [28]. Thus, the results of the various studies seem to have a limited generalizability. A meta-analysis of all clinical trials in NVAF patients may probably help to solve this problem [29]. Furthermore, this analysis should include echocardiographic data since these have been shown to be of considerable additional value in the selection of patients with a high risk of cerebral embolism [30].

In NVAF patients with recent TIA or stroke an additional risk factor might be the presence of coexistent, potentially causal arterial lesion of the extracranial arteries. As stated above, a proportion of fibrillating patients have concomitant arterial disease, which might have been the cause of the cerebral ischemic episode. Clinical criteria which help to identify emboli of cardiac origin in these patients are unreliable [31]. Furthermore, the finding of an arterial lesion which corresponds to the symptoms in a fibrillating patient does not automatically imply that it has been the cause of the cerebral ischemia. Whether concomitant cerebral vascular lesions are a risk factor or not remains to be established in the single secondary prevention study in NVAF patients, the European Atrial Fibrillation Trial (EAFT) [32].

What Is the Optimal Treatment to Prevent Embolism in NVAF?

The majority of earlier studies in patients with NVAF was non-randomized and uncontrolled [33]. Recently, however, the results of four randomized clinical trials have been published. In the Copenhagen AFASAK trial, 1,007 patients with nonvalvular AF were randomized to treatment with either anticoagulants, aspirin, or placebo [15]. The duration of treatment was 2 years or until the end of the study. Patients treated with anitcoagulation had a lower embolism rate than the other two groups. The numer of events was small, and – subsequently – the confidence limits were wide. Furthermore, neither the incidence of disabling events nor mortality were significantly reduced by anticoagulant treatment. The intention-to-treat analysis, which accounted for events that occurred after withdrawal of the study treatment, still showed a benefit from treatment with anticoagulation, but again, the confidence limits were very wide.

In 1990, the interim results of another primary trial, the North American Stroke Prevention in Atrial Fibrillation (SPAF) study, were published [16]. The preliminary results from this study showed a prevention of embolic events in patients who were treated with either anticoagulants or aspirin (the interim analysis did not provide the results of each of these two groups separately). This study showed that all patients who were treated with aspirin, including those who were not eligible for anticoagulation, had a lower rate of embolic complications than patients receiving placebo, but the confidence limits were very wide. The efficacy of aspirin was most marked in patients under the age of 70.

Also in 1990, the results of the Boston Area Anticoagulation Trial for Atrial Fibrillation (BAATAF) were published [17]. In this study, 420 patients were randomly allocated to treatment with anticoagulation or 'control treatment', which often included aspirin. This study showed a 86% (95% confidence limits, 51–96%) risk reduction by anticoaguation.

Finally, in the Canadian Atrial Fibrillation Anticoagulation (CAFA) study, 378 patients were randomized to double-blind treatment with anticoagulants or placebo [18]. The trial was stopped prematurely after the publication of the three other studies. The study showed a nonsignificant 37% (–64 to 76%) risk reduction by anticoagulation.

How Comparable Are Patients with NVAF Only and Patients with NVAF and Recent Cerebral Embolism?

Now that the four trials discussed above have shown unequivocal evidence that anticoagulation and aspirin are effective in the prevention of embolic complications in NVAF patients, the important issue is whether these results can be extrapolated to NVAF patients with a recent TIA or stroke. The answer to this pertinent question has to be provided by the EAFT in which NVAF patients with a recent TIA or minor stroke are randomized to anticoagulants, aspirin, or placebo. In May 1992, a total of 1,007 patients were randomized. The final results are expected in medio 1993. A preliminary comparison between the EAFT patients and those of the four primary prevention trials showed that there were no clear differences in baseline characteristics. The number of outcome events, however, was significantly different between the two populations: for stroke

7.5%/year versus 5%, for mortality 9%/year versus 4.5%. This may have important implications for the efficacy of both anticoagulation and aspirin.

How Comparable Are TIA or Stroke Patients with NVAF and Similar Patients with Sinus Rhythm?

Since various studies have shown the value of aspirin in patients with a TIA or minor stroke who have sinus rhythm [34], one may argue that aspirin is probably also effective in TIA or stroke patients with NVAF. Again, however, this conclusion is unsupported by clinical evidence. A comparison between NVAF patients entered into the EAFT and similar patients with sinus rhythm who were entered into another clinical trial, the Dutch TIA [35], shows a number of striking differences in baseline characteristics: NVAF patients are older, more often female, they have strokes rather than TIAs, less often smoke, have lower diastolic blood pressures and more often congestive heart disease than patients with sinus rhythm [36]. The CT scan shows that NVAF patients more often have an infarct, either symptomatic or not, and if symptomatic, the infarct is more often territorial or in borderzone areas, and less often small and deep [36]. Finally, the number of outcome events is significantly different between the two groups: for stroke 7.5%/year versus 6%, for mortality 9%/year versus 4%. All these differences show that one has to be cautious in extrapolating the results of previous aspirin studies in TIA or stroke patients to NVAF patients.

Conclusions

To conclude: (1) NVAF represents the most common cause of cardioembolic stroke. (2) Two-thirds of strokes in fibrillating patients are caused by embolism from the heart. (3) Patients with NVAF have an average risk of ischemic events of 5%/year; the risk depends on a number of clinical, and probably also, echocardiographic data. (4) Anticoagulation reduces the risk of embolism in NVAF patients by ± two-thirds (range 37–86%). (5) Aspirin has also been shown to be effective in NVAF patients, but the size of its benefit is unclear. (6) Patients with NVAF and a recent TIA or stroke have a much higher risk of ischemic events (7.5%/year) and a higher mortality (9%/year). (7) There are striking differences in clinical and CT findings between TIA/stroke patients with

AF and those with sinus rhythm. (8) The risk/benefit ratio of anticoagulants and aspirin in NVAF patients with a recent TIA or stroke is
uncertain.

Zusammenfassung

Nichtvalvuläres Vorhofflimmern und Schlaganfall

Die Inzidenz ischämischer zerebraler Insulte bei Patienten mit nichtvalvulärem Vor-
hofflimmern beträgt zwischen 2 und 5% im Jahr. Die Rezidivrate variiert in verschiedenen
Untersuchungen zwischen 2 und 15% innerhalb des ersten Jahres nach dem Schlaganfall.
Antikoagulantien reduzieren das Schlaganfallrisiko in der Primärprävention um etwa zwei
Drittel. Auch Acetylsalicylsäure ist prophylaktisch wirksam, allerdings ist der Grad der Ef-
fektivität derzeit noch nicht klar [Lancet 1989;i:175–178; N Engl J Med 1990;322:863–868;
N Engl J Med 1991;18:349–355; J Am Coll Cardiol 1991;18:349–355].

Bei einer Reihe von Schlaganfallpatienten mit Vorhofflimmern stellt sich die Frage, ob
die Rhythmusstörung tatsächlich als Ursache des Insults anzusehen ist oder nicht lediglich als
Hinweis auf eine fortgeschrittene generalisierte Arteriosklerose. Etwa 60% aller zerebralen
Insulte von Patienten mit Vorhofflimmern dürften tatsächlich Folge einer Embolie aus dem
Herzen sein [Arch Neurol 1986;43:71–84].

In einer Reihe von Untersuchungen konnten verschiedene Faktoren identifiziert werden, die das Risiko eines Schlaganfalls bei Vorhofflimmern erhöhen. Im einzelnen handelt es
sich um: weibliches Geschlecht, Alter, intermittierendes Vorhofflimmern, Größe des linken
Vorhofs, systolische und diastolische Hypertonie, früherer Myokardinfarkt, Angina pectoris,
Herzinsuffizienz und frühere Thromboembolien [Lancet 1987;i:526–529; Stroke
1989;20:1000–1004; Am J Cardiol 1989;63:366–367; Am J Cardiol 1990;65:1112–1116;
Arch Intern Med 1990;150:819–821; Ann Intern Med;116:1–5].

Seit kurzem liegen die Ergebnisse von 4 randomisierten Studien zur Primärprävention
von Embolien bei Vorhofflimmern vor. In der Kopenhagener AFASAK-Studie erhielten
1007 Patienten mit nichtvalvulärem Vorhofflimmern Antikoagulantien, Aspirin oder Plazebo. Die antikoagulatierten Patienten hatten eine niedrigere Embolierate als die Kranken der
anderen beiden Behandlungsgruppen. Allerdings wurde weder die Inzidenz schwerer Embolien noch die Letalität durch Antikoagulation signifikant gesenkt. Die Ergebnisse der amerikanischen SPAF-Studie zeigten, daß sowohl Antikoagulantien als auch Aspirin einen präven-
tiven Effekt haben [N Engl J Med 1990;322:863–868]. In einer weiteren amerikanischen
Untersuchung (BAATAF) erhielten 420 Patienten entweder Antikoagulantien oder eine
«Kontrollbehandlung», die oftmals Acetylsalicylsäure umfaßte. Die Studie zeigte eine
Risikoreduktion embolischer Ereignisse um 86% durch Antikoagulation [N Engl J Med
1991;18:349–355]. Eine kanadische Studie (CAFA) wurde nach Publikation der Ergebnisse
der genannten Untersuchungen abgebrochen [J Am Coll Cardiol 1991;18:349–355].

Offen ist die Frage, ob die Ergebnisse dieser Primärpräventionsstudien auch übertragen
werden können auf Patienten, die bereits einen ischämischen Insult bei Vorhofflimmern erlitten haben. Der Frage der effektivsten Sekundärprävention wurde nachgegangen in einer mul-
tizentrischen europäischen Untersuchungsreihe (EAFT), deren endgültige Ergebnisse 1993
erwartet werden.

References

1   Kannel WB, Abbott RD, Savage DD, McNamara PM: Epidemiologic features of chronic atrial fibrillation: The Framingham Study. N Engl J Med 1982;306:1018–1022.

2   Martin A: Atrial fibrillation in the elderly. Br Med J 1977;i:712–716.

3   Olsson SB: Atrial fibrillation – Some current problems. Acta Med Scand 1980;207:2–4.

4   Sherman DG, Goldman L, Whiting RB, et al: Risk of thrombo-embolism in patients with atrial fibrillation. Arch Neurol 1986;43:68–70.

5   Wolf PA, Darsber TR, Thomas HE: Epidemiologic assessment of chronic atrial fibrillation and risk of stroke: The Framingham Study. Neurology 1983;28:973–977.

6   Harrison MJG, Marshall J: Atrial fibrillation, TIAs and completed stroke. Stroke 1984;15:441–442.

7   Bogousslavsky J, Hechinski VC, Boughner DR, et al: Cardiac lesions and arterial lesions in carotid transient ischemic attacks. Arch Neurol 1986;43:223–228.

8   Koudstaal PJ, van Gijn J, Klootwijk APJ, et al: Holter monitoring in patients with transient and focal ischemic attacks of the brain. Stroke 1986;17:192–195.

9   Fisher CM: Reducing risks of cerebral embolism. Geriatrics 1979;34:59–66.

10   Flegel KM, Shipley MJ, Rose G: Risk of stroke in non-rheumatic atrial fibrillation. Lancet 1987;i:526–529.

11   Kopecky SL, Gersh BJ, McGoon MD, et al: The natural history of lone atrial fibrillation. N Engl J Med 1987;317:669–674.

12   Sage JL, Van Uitert RL: Risk of recurrent stroke with atrial fibrillation: Differences between rheumatic and arteriosclerotic heart disease. Stroke 1980;14:537–540.

13   Wolf PA, Kannel WB, McGee DL; et al: Duration of atrial fibrillation and imminence of stroke: The Framingham Study. Stroke 1983;14:664–667.

14   Cerebral Embolism Task Force: Cardiogenic brain embolism. Arch Neurol 1986;43:71–84.

15   Petersen P, Boysen G, Godtfredsen J, Andersen ED, Andersen B: Placebo-controlled, randomised trial of warfarin and aspirin for prevention of thromboembolic complications in chronic atrial fibrillation. Lancet 1989;i:175–178.

16   Stroke Prevention in Atrial Fibrillation Study Group Investigators: Preliminary report of the Stroke Prevention in Atrial Fibrillation Study. N Engl J Med 1990;322:863–868.

17   The Bosten Area Anticoagulation Trial for Atrial Fibrillation Investigators: The effect of low-dose warfarin on the risk of stroke in patients with nonrheumatic atrial fibrillation. N Engl J Med 1990;323:1505–1511.

18   Connolly SJ, Laupacis A, Gent M, Roberts RS, Cairns JA, Joyner C, for the CAFA Study Coinvestigators: Canadian Atrial Fibrillation Anticoagulation (CAFA) Study. J Am Coll Cardiol 1991;18:349–355.

19   Castaigne P, Lhermitte F, Gautier JC, et al: Internal carotid artery occlusion – A study of 61 instances in 50 patients with postmortem data. Brain 1970;93:231–258.

20   Brand FN, Abbott RD, Kannal WB, Wolf PA: Characteristics of lone atrial fibrillation – 30 years follow-up in the Framingham Study. J Am Med Assoc 1985;284:3449–3459.

21   Britton M, Gustafson C: Nonrheumatic atrial fibrillation as a risk factor for stroke. Stroke 1985;16:182–188.

22   Jörgensen L, Torvik A: Ischemic cerebrovascular disease in an autopsy series. J Neurol Sci 1966;3:490–509.

23   Cerebral Embolism Task Force: Cardiogenic brain embolism. Arch Neurol 1986;43:71–84.
24   Flegel KM, Hanley J: Risk factors for stroke and other embolic events in patients with nonrheumatic atrial fibrillation. Stroke 1989;20:1000–1004.
25   Aronow WS, Gutstein H, Hsieh FY: Risk factors for thromboembolic stroke in elderly patients with chronic atrial fibrillation. Am J Cardiol 1989;63:366–367.
26   Cabin HS, Clubb KS, Hall C, Perlmutter RA, Feinstein AR: Risk for systemic embolization of atrial fibrillation without mitral stenosis. Am J Cardiol 1990;65:1112–1116.
27   Petersen P; Kastrup J, Helweg-Larsen S, Boysen G, Godtfredsen J: Risk factors for thromboembolic complications in chronic atrial fibrillation. Arch Intern Med 1990;150:819–821.
28   The Stroke Prevention in Atrial Fibrillation Investigators: Predictors of thomboembolism in atrial fibrillation. I. Clinical features of patients at risk. Ann Intern Med 1992;116:1–5.
29   Walker MD: Atrial fibrillation und antithrombotic prophylaxis, a prospective meta-analyses. Lancet 1989;i:325–326.
30   The Stroke Prevention in Atrial Fibrillation Investigators: Predictors of thromboembolism in atrial fibrillation. II. Echocardiographic features of patients at risk. Ann Intern Med 1992;116:6–12.
31   Britton M, Gustafsson C: Nonrheumatic atrial fibrillation as a risk factor for stroke. Stroke 1985;16:182–188.
32   The European Atrial Fibrillation Trial Study Group: The European Atrial Fibrillation Trial – The secondary preventive effect of anticoagulants and of acetylsalicylic acid in patients with non-rheumatic atrial fibrillation and a TIA or non-disabling stroke. Study protocol, January 1990.
33   Koudstaal PJ: Stroke prevention in non-valvular atrial fibrillation. Some methodological aspects; in Amery WK, Bousser M-G, Clifford Rose F (eds): Clinical Trial Methodology in Stroke. London, Baillière Tindall, 1989;pp:239–247.
34   Antiplatelet Trialists Collaboration: Secondary prevention of vascular disease by prolonged antiplatelet treatment. Br Med J 1988;296:320–331.
35   The Dutch TIA Trial Study Group: A comparison of two doses of aspirin (30 vs. 283 mg/day) in patients after a transient ischemic attack or minor ischemic stroke. N Engl J Med 1991;325:1261–1266.
36   Van Latum JC, Koudstaal PJ, van Gijn J, Algra A, for the European Atrial Fibrillation Trial and Dutch TIA Study Group: A comparison of baseline characteristics in patients with a TIA or minor stroke and with or without nonvalvular atrial fibrillation (in preparation).
37   Van Latum JC, Koudstaal PJ, van Gijn J, Algra A, for the European Atrial Fibrillation Trial and Dutch TIA Study Group: A comparison of CT scan findings in TIA or minor stroke patients, with or without nonvalvular atrial fibrillation (in preparation).

Peter. J. Koudstaal, MD
Department of Neurology
University Hospital Rotterdam
Academisch Ziekenhuis Dijkzigt
40 Dr. Molewaterplein
NL–3015 GD Rotterdam (The Netherlands)

Dorndorf W, Marx P (eds): Stroke Prevention.
Basel, Karger, 1994, pp 188–196

Prevention of Cardioembolic Stroke

G. Boysen[a], P. Petersen[a], J. Godtfredsen[b]

[a] Department of Neurology, Rigshospitalet, and [b] Department of Cardiology,
Herlev Hospital, Copenhagen, Denmark

Prevention of stroke in cardiac diseases usually is a secondary object, while prevention of acute myocardial infarction (AMI) and cardiac death is the primary aim of therapeutical intervention. Often, however, antithrombotic therapy has an effect on all three types of events. It has therefore in many studies become customary to lump the three vascular events together and to consider the combined risk reduction obtained by a given treatment.

Almost all types of heart diseases are associated with increased risk of stroke, either due to thromboembolism from the heart, or because of hypertension or a more widespread atherosclerotic vascular disease that affects both the brain and the heart.

At the same time as treatment of AMI has undergone a revolution by the convincing results of thrombolysis therapy [1], anticoagulation therapy has experienced a renaissance as prophylactic treatment of thromboembolic events in atrial fibrillation [2] as well as after AMI [3]. The effect of antiplatelet therapy in the prevention of serious cardiovascular events, documented in numerous trials, has been subject to overview analysis [4] establishing valid estimates of its effect in various cardiovascular diseases. Trials aiming at evaluating whether anticoagulation therapy is more effective than the far cheaper and more easily controlled aspirin treatment are underway or in the planning phase. New strategies with different levels of intensity of anticoagulation therapy, and with a combination of anticoagulation and antiplatelet therapy are developed.

Stratification of Thromboembolic Risk

Stein et al. [5] classified various clinical heart disease syndromes into three levels of thromboembolic risk (table 1). Conditions with a risk of thromboembolic events greater than 6%/year were considered high risk. The intermediate group had a risk of 2–6%/year, and the lowest level had a risk of thromboembolic events below 2%/year. For comparison, individuals without signs of cardiac disease carry a risk of thromboembolic events below 1%/year.

Patients in the high-risk group require intensive antithrombotic therapy; the intermediate group requires less intensive treatment, while treatment in the low-risk group may be of questionable value. The thromboembolic events considered here include AMI, systemic embolism, vascular death, and stroke. The relative frequency of these events varies with the various disease entities. For instance, in atrial fibrillation, cerebrovascular events constitute more than 80% of all events, while following AMI, reinfarction and death are the most common events. The important relation

Table 1. Thromboembolism in cardiac disease based on pathogenesis and risk

Pathogenesis	Thromboembolic risk		
	high (>6%/year)	medium (2–6%/year)	low (<2%/year)
Arterial system Platelets + fibrin	unstable angina acute MI after thrombolysis PTCA–early phase SVBG–early phase	chronic stable angina chronic phase after MI PTCA–chronic phase SVBG–chronic phase	primary prevention of cardiovascular disease
Cardiac chambers Fibrin	A-fib–prior embolism A-fib–mitral stenosis	A-fib–other forms of organic heart disease; early phase after anterior MI dilated cardiomyopathy	A-fib–idiopathic chronic LV aneurysm
Prosthetic valves Fibrin + platelets	old mechanical prostheses mechanical prostheses – prior embolism	recent mechanical prostheses bioprostheses–A-fib	bioprostheses–normal sinus rhythm

MI = Myocardial infarction; PTCA = percutaneous transluminal coronary angioplasty; SVBG = saphenous vein bypass graft; A-fib = atrial fibrillation; LV = left ventricular.

between the heart and the brain calls for cooperation between specialists across medical disciplines.

The following discussion will be confined to two heart disease syndromes: AMI and atrial fibrillation with respect to risk of thrombo-embolism and the prevention thereof.

Acute Myocardial Infarction

In the acute phase of AMI the risk of stroke is modest compared to the risk of reinfarction and cardiac death; however, the ISIS-2 study [1] showed a significant reduction of stroke occurrence by aspirin 160 mg daily during the first month after AMI.

Chronic Phase after AMI

Patients in the chronic phase after AMI belong to the intermediate risk group. Antiplatelet therapy, according to an overview analysis [4], reduced the risk of vascular death by 13%, nonfatal AMI by 31% and nonfatal stroke by 42%. The risk of vascular death within the observation period was 7 times greater than the risk of stroke.

Whether anticoagulation therapy in the post-AMI phase is superior to aspirin therapy is still an open question. International Anticoagulation Review Group [6] showed in 1970 that anticoagulation therapy reduced the mortality after AMI by 20%. A recent Norwegian study [3], in which 1,214 patients were randomized to anticoagulation therapy with warfarin or placebo in a double-blind fashion, showed a 24% reduction in mortality, 43% reduction in nonfatal AMI and 61% reduction in cerebrovascular events in the warfarin-treated patients. Thus, it seems as if anticoagulation is more effective, but a direct comparison is still lacking.

Atrial Fibrillation

The prevalence of atrial fibrillation in Copenhagen, Denmark [7], was recently found to be 1% in the age group 60–70 years, 3% in the age group 70–80 years, and above 4% in the age group 80 years or older, equal in the two sexes (table 2). The yearly stroke incidence in patients with nonval-

Table 2. Prevalence of atrial fibrillation in the Copenhagen City Heart Study 1976–83

Age	F	M
60–64	0.4	1.2
65–69	1.1	1.2
70–74	3.1	2.2
75–79	3.1	4.1
80–	4.1	4.3

vular atrial fibrillation ranges from 3 to 8%, which is substantially higher than the stroke incidence in the general population of similar age. Atrial fibrillation is found in 13–15% of stroke patients.

Paroxysmal atrial fibrillation carries a lower risk of stroke than chronic atrial fibrillation, as shown by Petersen and Godtfredsen [8] and Treseder et al. [9], who found the risk below 2%/year.

Causes of Atrial Fibrillation

The underlying heart diseases in chronic nonvalvular atrial fibrillation are hypertensive heart disease, coronary heart disease, congestive heart failure, and cardiomyopathy. Thyrotoxicosis, a noncardiac cause of atrial fibrillation, is important to recognize, because treatment may result in conversion to lasting sinus rhythm [10]. The prevalence of the various conditions varies from one study to another. In some patients no cardiac cause of atrial fibrillation is discernible, and this condition is called lone or idiopathic atrial fibrillation. The prevalence of lone atrial fibrillation among atrial fibrillation patients varies considerably among studies. When using strict criteria as Godtfredsen [11] or Kopecky et al. [12] the prevalence is about or below 2–3% of atrial fibrillation patients. The risk of stroke is low in lone atrial fibrillation (table 1).

Antithrombotic Therapy in Atrial Fibrillation

In atrial fibrillation due to valvular disease or to rheumatic heart disease, the risk of stroke is high, and several smaller studies have suggested anticoagulation therapy as the prophylactic treatment of choice [for references, see 13].

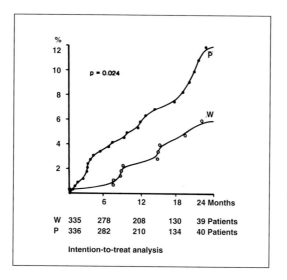

Fig. 1. Copenhagen AFASAK Study. Cumulative rate of thromboembolic events in 335 patients randomized to anticoagulation therapy with warfarin (W) compared to 336 patients randomized to placebo (P) evaluated by intention-to-treat analysis.

Patients with nonvalvular atrial fibrillation, who have already had a cerebrovascular event, constitute a high-risk group with event rate of about 10%/year, highest in the early phase after an event. The Cerebral Embolism Study Group [14] recommended anticoagulation therapy in this patient group. However, the study included few patients, and there is not yet agreement as to the best preventive strategy in such patients. The ongoing European Atrial Fibrillation Trial [15] is a secondary prevention study in patients with atrial fibrillation who have had a recent transient ischemic attack or a minor stroke. It evaluates the effect of anticoagulation versus aspirin versus placebo.

In patients with nonvalvular atrial fibrillation without prior cerebrovascular event, four independent studies of stroke prophylaxis have been completed: the Copenhagen AFASAK Study [2], in which AF stands for atrial fibrillation, AS for aspirin and AK for anticoagulation (fig. 1), the Stroke Prevention in Atrial Fibrillation Study (SPAF) [16], the Boston Area Anticoagulation Trial for Atrial Fibrillation (BAATAF) [17], and the Canadian Atrial Fibrillation Anticoagulation Study (CAFA) [18]. The four trials comprise a total of 1,890 patients randomized to either anticoagulation or placebo. The absolute stroke risk was 4.4%/year in the placebo group and 1.5%/year in the warfarin group. The risk reduction of 66% is highly statistically significant. A fifth study, the Stroke Prevention in Nonvalvular Atrial Fibrillation (SPINAF), has been completed, but not yet published. The BAATAF Study [17] found a significantly lower mortality among warfarin-treated patients. A cooperative working group from the five studies is preparing a combined analysis of the overall effect on stroke, systemic emboli and mortality as well as an analysis of risk factors for stroke among atrial fibrillation patients.

The dreaded risk of anticoagulation therapy is intracranial hemorrhage, which in these studies occurred at a frequency of 0.3%/year in the warfarin group compared to a frequency below 0.1% in the placebo group [19]. Other major bleeding episodes were below 1%/year and equally frequent in both treatment groups, while minor bleeding episodes were more common in the warfarin group (5.0 vs. 1.5%).

The optimal therapeutic range for oral anticoagulation has not been established. However, the target range for BAATAF and CAFA was International Normalized Ratio (INR) values of 1.5–3.0, which indicates that low intensity anticoagulation may give sufficient prevention against thromboembolic events from the heart. The effectiveness of low intensity anticoagulation therapy was evidenced by a risk reduction of 86% in the BAATAF Study, i e. higher than that found in the other studies.

The Role of Aspirin in Nonvalvular Atrial Fibrillation

Two of the above studies, the AFASAK [2] and SPAF-I [16] evaluated the effect of aspirin on thromboembolic events. In the AFASAK Study, 336 patients were treated with aspirin 75 mg daily, and in SPAF-I, 552 patients received 325 mg aspirin daily. In the AFASAK Study the effect of aspirin was not statistically different from that of placebo, while the SPAF-I study found a risk reduction of 42%. One possible explanation for the different results in the two studies is that the median age was 74 years in the AFASAK Study and 67 years in the SPAF Study. Whether the different doses of aspirin play a role is unclear and less probable, since an aspirin dose of 75 mg daily in the RISC Study [20] was highly effective in reducing the risk of AMI and death in patients with unstable angina. It is possible that the difference is a result of the play of chance, and that the small and insignificant risk reduction in the AFASAK Study falls within the confidence limits of that of the SPAF Study.

Conclusion

Prevention of stroke in cardiac diseases usually is obtained by means of the same therapy that prevents acute myocardial infarction and cardiac death. Cardiac diseases can be stratified into three levels of risk of thromboembolism. A yearly risk above 6% constitutes the high-risk group, a risk of 2–6% the intermediate group, and below 2% the low-risk group. In the chronic phase after AMI, stroke prevention may be obtained by platelet inhibitory drugs as well as by anticoagulation therapy. In chronic nonvalvular atrial fibrillation a low intensity anticoagulation aiming at INR values of 1.5–3.0 reduces stroke risk by 60–70%. Aspirin has been shown also to have some stroke-preventive effect in nonvalvular atrial fibrillation.

Zusammenfassung

Prävention kardioembolischer Insulte

Praktisch alle Herzerkrankungen sind mit einem erhöhten Hirninfarktrisiko verbunden. Stein et al. [Circulation 1989;80:1501] klassifizierten verschiedene Herzerkrankungen nach ihrem Embolierisiko in 3 Kategorien:

Hohes Risiko (>6% pro Jahr): instabile Angina pectoris; akuter Myokardinfarkt; nach Thrombolyse; Frühphase nach PTCA; Frühphase nach aorto-koronarem Bypass; Vorhofflimmern mit eingetretenem Insult; Vorhofflimmern mit Mitralstenose; mechanische Klappenprothese alten Typs; mechanische Klappenprothese mit eingetretenem Insult. *Mittleres Risiko* (2–6% pro Jahr): chronische, stabile Angina pectoris; chronische Phase nach Myokardinfarkt; chronische Phase nach PTCA; chronische Phase nach aorto-koronarem Bypass; Vorhofflimmern mit anderen organischen Herzerkrankungen; Frühphase nach Vorderwandinfarkt; dilatative Kardiomyophatie; mechanische Klappenprothese neuer Bauart; biologische Klappenprothese und Vorhofflimmern. *Niedriges Risiko* (<2% pro Jahr): Primärprävention kardiovaskulärer Erkrankungen; idiopathisches Vorhofflimmern; chronisches linksventrikuläres Aneurysma; biologische Klappenprothese bei Sinusrhythmus.

Patienten mit hohem Risiko sollten intensiv antithrombotisch behandelt werden. Bei mittlerem Risiko reicht eine weniger intensive Therapie aus. Der Nutzen einer Antikoagulation bei Patienten mit niedrigem Risiko ist fraglich.

Zwei besondere Probleme, Myokardinfarkt und Vorhofflimmern, sollen im folgenden gesondert diskutiert werden.

In der *akuten Phase des Myokardinfarktes* ist das Hirninfarktrisiko zwar deutlich erhöht, jedoch deutlich geringer als das des Herztodes oder eines kardialen Reinfarktes. ISIS 2 [Lancet 1988;ii:349–360] hat eine signifikante Schlaganfallsreduktion durch 160 mg ASS nachgewiesen.

In der *chronischen Phase nach Myokardinfarkt* reduziert ASS nach den Ergebnissen einer Metaanalyse [Br Med J 1988;296:320–331] vaskuläre Todesfälle um 13%, nichttödliche Myokardinfarkte um 31% und nichttödliche Hirninfarkte um 42%.

Ob eine Antikoagulation in der Postmyokardinfarktphase der Antiaggregation mit ASS überlegen ist, läßt sich aufgrund des Fehlens von direkten Vergleichsstudien nicht sagen. In einer Norwegischen Untersuchung [N Engl J Med 1990;323:147–152] reduzierte Warfarin die Sterblichkeit gegenüber Plazebo um 24%, nicht-tödliche Myokardinfarkte um 42% und zerebrale ischämische Insulte um 61%.

Vorhofflimmern findet sich in Kopenhagen, Dänemark, bei 60–70jährigen in 1%, bei 70–80jährigen in 3% und bei Einwohnern über 80 Jahren in 4%. Ursachen chronischen Vorhofflimmerns sind hypertensive und koronare Herzerkrankungen, Herzinsuffizienz, Kardiomyopathien und Hyperthyreose. Idiopathisches Vorhofflimmern wird bei Kranken ohne die genannten Grundkrankheiten diagnostiziert.

Vorhofflimmern bei rheumatischen oder nichtrheumatischen Klappenfehlern ist mit hohem Embolierisiko verbunden und sollte mit Antikoagulantien behandelt werden [J Neurol Neurosurg Psychiatry 1974;37:378–383].

Wegen des hohen Insultrisikos gilt dies auch für die Sekundärprophylaxe bei Patienten mit *Vorhofflimmern ohne Klappenfehler.* Ob ASS hier eine der Antikoagulation vergleichbare Wirksamkeit in der Sekundärprophylaxe ischämischer Insulte hat, ist Gegenstand des noch nicht abgeschlossenen European Atrial Fibrillation Trial.

In der *Primärprophylaxe ischämischer Insulte bei nichtvalvulärem Vorhofflimmern* haben 4 Untersuchungen [Lancet 1989;i:175–179, Stroke Prevention in Atrial Fibrillation Study Group Investigators (SPAF), N Engl J Med 1990;333:863–868; The Boston Area Anticoagulation Trial for Atrial Fibrillation Investigators (BAATAF), N Engl J Med 1990;322:1505–1511; Canadian Atrial Fibrillation Antikoagulation Study (CAFA) JACC 1991;18:349–355] übereinstimmend eine Schlaganfallreduktion um etwa 66% durch Antikoagulation mit Warfarin nachgewiesen (Schlaganfallsrate Plazebo 4,4%/Jahr, Warfarin 1,5%/Jahr). Intrakranielle Blutungen ereigneten sich unter Plazebo in <0,1%/Jahr, unter Warfarin in 0,3%/Jahr. Die optimale Warfarindosis ist bisher nicht eindeutig bekannt. BAATAF und CAFA benutzten einen niedrigen INR(International Normalized Ratio)-Wert von 1,5–3,0, so daß eine Wirksamkeit auch bei niedriger Dosierung erwiesen ist.

Ob ASS wirksam ist, läßt sich zur Zeit noch nicht eindeutig sagen. Der Effekt von 75 mg ASS/Tag zeigte in AFASAK keinen statistischen Unterschied zu Placebo, während 325 mg ASS/Tag in SPAF I eine Risikominderung um 42% bewirkten. Ob dieser Unterschied durch die unterschiedlichen Dosen oder durch andere Faktoren bedingt ist, muß zur Zeit offen bleiben.

References

1   ISIS-2 (Second International Study of Infarct Survival) Collaborative Group: Randomised trial of intravenous streptokinase, oral aspirin, both, or neither among 17, 187 cases of suspected acute myocardial infarction. Lancet 1988;ii:349–360.

2   Petersen P, Boysen G, Godtfredsen J, Andersen ED, Andersen B: Placebo-controlled, randomised trial of warfarin and aspirin for prevention of thromboembolic complications in chronic atrial fibrillation. The Copenhagen AFASAK Study. Lancet 1989,i:175–179.

3   Smith P, Arnesen H, Holme I: The effect of warfarin on mortality and reinfarction after myocardial infarction. N Engl J Med 1990;323:147–152.

4   Antiplatelet Trialists' Collaboration: Secondary prevention of vascular disease by prolonged antiplatelet treatment. Br Med J 1988;296:320–331.

5   Stein B, Fuster V, Halperin JL, Chesebro JH: Antithrombotic therapy in cardiac disease. An emerging approach based on pathogenesis and risk. Circulation 1989;80:1501–1513.

6   International Anticoagulant Review Group: Collaborative analysis of long-term anticoagulation administration after acute myocardial infarction. Lancet 1970;i:203–209.

7   The Copenhagen City Heart Study: Østerbroundersøgelsen. A book of tables with data from the first examination (1976–78) and a five-year follow-up (1981–83). Scand J Soc Med 1989;17: suppl 41.

8   Petersen P, Godtfredsen J: Embolic complications in paroxysmal atrial fibrillation. Stroke 1986;17:622–626.

9   Treseder AS, Sastry BSD, Thomas TPL, Yates MA, Pathy MSJ: Atrial fibrillation and stroke in elderly hospitalized patients. Age Ageing 1986;15:89–92.

10 Petersen P, Hansen JM: Stroke in thyrotoxicosis with atrial fibrillation. Stroke 1988;19:15–18.

11 Godtfredsen J: Atrial Fibrillation. Etiology, Course and Prognosis. A Follow-Up Study of 1,212 Cases. Copenhagen, Munksgaard, 1975.

12 Kopecky SL, Gersh BJ, McGoon MD, Whisnant JP, Holmes DR, Ilstrup DM, Frye RL: The natural history of lone atrial fibrillation: A population-based study over three decades. N Engl J Med 1987;317:669–674.

13 Adams GF, Merrett JD, Hutchinson WM, Pollock AM: Cerebral embolism and mitral stenosis: Survival with and without anticoagulants. J Neurol Neurosurg Psychiatry 1974;37:378–383.

14 Cerebral Embolism Study Group: Immediate anticoagulation of embolic stroke: A randomized trial. Stroke 1983;14:668–676.

15 Walker MD: Atrial fibrillation and antithrombotic prophylaxis: A prospective meta-analysis. Lancet 1989;i:325–326.

16 Stroke Prevention in Atrial Fibrillation Study Group Investigators: Preliminary report of the stroke prevention in atrial fibrillation study. N Engl J Med 1990;322:863–868.

17 The Boston Area Anticoagulation Trial for Atrial Fibrillation Investigators: The effect of low-dose warfarin on the risk of stroke in patients with nonrheumatic atrial fibrillation. N Engl J Med 1990;323:1505–1511.

18 Connolly SJ, Laupacis A, Gent M, Roberts RS, Cairns JA, Joyner C for the CAFA Study Coinvestigators: Canadian Atrial Fibrillation Anticoagulation (CAFA) Study. J Am Coll Cardiol 1991;18:349–355.

19 Albers GW, Sherman DG, Gress DR, Paulseth JE, Petersen P: Stroke prevention in nonvalvular atrial fibrillation: A review of prospective randomized trials. Ann Neurol 1991;30:511–518.

20 The RISC Group: Risk of myocardial infarction and death during treatment with low dose aspirin and intravenous heparin in men with unstable coronary artery disease. Lancet 1990;336:827–830.

Gudrun Boysen, MD, DMSc,
Department of Neurology
Hvidovre Hospital, University Copenhagen
DK-2650 Copenhagen (Denmark)

Subject Index